P9-AQL-600

# Walk Your Way Through Menopause

CHICAGO PUBLIC LIBRARY
WEST ENGLEWOOD BRANCH
1745 W. 63rd STREET
CHICAGO, IL  60636

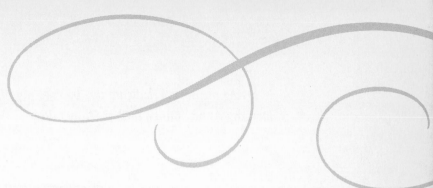

# Walk Your Way Through Menopause

14 Programs to Get in Shape,

Boost Your Mood, and Recharge Your Sex Life

No Matter What Your Current Fitness Level

## Maggie Spilner

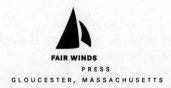

**FAIR WINDS**
PRESS
GLOUCESTER, MASSACHUSETTS

*In loving memory, I dedicate this book to my mother,*
*Dorothy Anne Spilner, and my father, Robert Walker Spilner.*

Text © 2005 by Maggie Spilner

First published in the USA in 2005 by
Fair Winds Press
33 Commercial Street
Gloucester, MA 01930

All rights reserved. No part of this book may be reproduced or utilized, in any form or by any means, electronic or mechanical, without prior permission in writing from the publisher.

09 08 07 06 05   1 2 3 4 5

ISBN 1-59233-129-7

Library of Congress Cataloging-in-Publication Data available

Cover design by Mary Ann Smith
Book design by Leslie Haimes
Illustrations by Nicole Kaufman

Printed and bound in Canada

The information in this book is for educational purposes only. It is not intended to replace the advice of a physician or medical practitioner. Please see your health care provider before beginning any new health program.

# Contents

THE CHICAGO PUBLIC LIBRARY
*WEST ENGLEWOOD BRANCH*
1745 W. 63RD STREET
CHICAGO ILLINOIS 60636
312-747-3481

R03123 74963

SEP    2006

*T*his book is for women who are beginning to realize that taking a daily walk may be one of, if not *the* best, safest, most convenient, and most effective tools they have to combat some of the conditions associated with the withdrawal and eventual loss of estrogen and the effects of aging. It's not a source of medical information, but a series of programs designed to help you stay motivated and inspired for the rest of your life. The workbook format allows you to keep records of the various programs you try. Hopefully you will come back to it again and again, whenever you find yourself slacking off, bored or itching for something new. You may find, as I did, that no single program can satisfy you for long, and you will develop your own multi-dimensional walking style that draws from many of these programs.

Menopause was not a dreadful transition for me. One year after my final period, I found myself wondering what the big deal was. If anything, I felt more stable, emotionally, than ever before. Perhaps part of the reason I weathered it well was that I had been exercising consistently since my early thirties, and continued to exercise during the transition. It signals a time of life that is unencumbered by body processes that are sometimes painful, emotionally trying, or inconvenient. I entered a whole new life, both in career and attitude. For me, my fifties are an entirely new beginning. The same may well be true for you. I hope that you enter this phase of life looking forward to new horizons, and that you are willing to take the time to care for yourself by beginning or continuing to exercise regularly. Here's an Irish blessing I recently came across. It offers just the right touch of spirit and laughter to accompany you on your mid-life walks through  menopause and beyond. I send it your way with a smile!

—*Maggie*

*May the light always find you on a dreary day.*
*When you need to be home, may you find your way.*
*May you always have courage to take a chance*
*And never find frogs in your underpants.*

# Introduction

*I* knew my mother had suffered a hot flash one day when I came home from high school and found the living room furniture completely reconfigured. It seems counterintuitive—all that pushing and shoving when you feel you ought to be taking a cold shower—but my mother suffered from anxiety attacks, and to her, hot flashes felt a lot like panic creeping up on her. Her solution to panic, and thus to hot flashes, was to get moving! She took her mind off her symptoms and used the power of her hormonal surge to move the sofa.

That's about all I learned from my mother about menopause. Of course, I wasn't particularly interested in knowing any more at the time. I just remember her laughing about it. My mom tried to laugh about a lot of things that bothered her. She had a little blackboard in the kitchen, and one day she wrote on it, "If life gives you lemons, make lemonade!" It stayed there for a decade.

Meanwhile, if night sweats disturbed her sleep, I would never have noticed. She often worked on her oil paintings well into the night, after we were all in bed. Both my parents were night owls, watching late-night TV, reading, or painting. In fact, one night I waited, fully clothed under the sheets, for my parents to go to sleep so that I could meet a classmate I knew was waiting for me outside with a thermos of hot chocolate, ready for an adventurous walk around town in the middle of the night. But my parents never went to bed!

Neither my sisters nor I know whether or not my mother used estrogen. My mother wasn't big on doctors and did not see even one during the ten years after my dad passed away, which is when we became more involved in knowing about her health care. She completely avoided breast exams and Pap smears. When she began to show signs of dementia in her late seventies, the doctor we dragged her to tried estrogen as therapy. But it caused irregular bleeding, so we stopped it.

My mother passed away six months after her eightieth birthday, when I was fifty. I was already well through menopause by then, but we never discussed it. Of course, now I wish that I had asked more about her history. I started having perimenopausal symptoms in my late thirties—very heavy bleeding, mostly. By about forty-two or forty-three, I was having occasional hot flashes. They never bothered me much. I was much more bothered by the fact that I had to start wearing reading glasses! At forty-five, I went on a hiking tour to Austria for a week. A couple of months after I returned, I realized I hadn't had a period since before I left. I went to see my doctor and she said, "You're too young to be menopausal. Your body is probably just reacting to the overseas flight." A couple of months later, I called to say that I still hadn't had a period, and she sent me for a blood test. The test revealed that I had almost no estrogen in my body. My doctor seemed shocked, but I wasn't. We then realized that my recurrent vaginal problems (itching and burning sensations and painful intercourse) were actually the result of menopausal changes: thinning membranes, less lubrication, shortening of the vagina. We also figured out that the overall sense of "flatness" that had been bothering me for about a year was probably the result of "estrogen withdrawal." I did experience more hot flashes at night (called night sweats) and would drive my husband crazy throwing off the covers one moment and tucking them up around my chin the next. The sleep disturbances were annoying, but not particularly draining. I got used to waking up, removing the covers, and falling back to sleep again.

Because of the night sweats and the vaginal problems, I asked my doctor if I should try hormone replacement therapy (HRT). It seemed to be the thing to do. Estrogen was being touted as something of a miracle drug that not only relieved annoying menopausal symptoms but also protected women from future problems with osteoporosis and heart disease. Researchers suggested that estrogen could help us stay younger looking by helping to keep our skin supple, thick, and wrinkle-free longer. (Maybe that was the most tempting idea of all!) According to everything I'd read up to that point, it seemed smart to give it a try.

I knew that I was a lousy pill taker. So I asked for an estrogen patch, which I wore on my belly. That lasted about two months. I can't really explain what it was, but I just didn't feel right. I ended up dumping the patch and taking a form of the herb black cohosh, called Remifemin. This herb has been approved in Germany for the treatment of menopausal symptoms. I took the lowest possible dose known to be effective and found the herb worked wonders for my vaginal problems and also seemed to be something of a mood elevator (which I discovered later was also one of its reported benefits). The night sweats subsided over time. After about a year, I stopped taking the herbal supplement.

But all the hoopla around HRT made me feel like I'd really be missing out on an important preventive medicine by deciding not to take estrogen. I was a daily exerciser, but books and magazines I read, including the one I worked for, seemed to be suggesting that HRT was a key player in protection from future heart attacks and thinning bones. I'd spent the last ten years writing about the benefits of exercise to your heart, your bones, your brain—every aspect of your health. So why HRT? Was the research directed at women who rarely exercise? Was it more promotion than science?

My doctor agreed that my devotion to regular exercise was probably more important than taking estrogen. In fact, she was conservative in her prescription of it. She would not recommend anyone stay on estrogen therapy for more than six months, because she believed we just didn't know enough about its long-term consequences. How right she was. Seven years later, studies have shown that estrogen not only doesn't protect against heart disease, it may contribute to it. The use of HRT has now been related to heart disease, stroke, cancer, and even Alzheimer's. What once looked like a miracle drug now looks like a medical disaster for some women. While HRT is still being recommended by many doctors for menopausal symptoms, many women are seeking other alternatives, both for easing their perimenopausal symptoms and protecting their health after menopause.

# Chapter One

# Menopause and the Benefits of Exercise

*"What is the first thing I should do to age successfully? Walk."*

—David Snowdon PhD, Aging With Grace

Menopause. A word rarely mentioned in most households fifty years ago is out of the closet—way out. There's even a musical about it. (It's called *Menopause: The Musical* and it has been performed all over the country). Baby Boomer women, who have driven the marketplace for a generation and are now in the midst of midlife, have made "the change" (as our mothers called it) a common topic in books, magazines, and radio and TV talk shows. Boomer women, not willing to accept *any* change lying down, have taken a proactive approach to menopause, challenging prevailing attitudes and behaviors. Hot flashes, reframed as "power surges," have become symbols of energy and, if not desirable, are at least less embarrassing. We can joke about it, even in public, and in front of the men in our lives.

But just because we're laughing doesn't mean we're not concerned. Just the opposite. Our generation has been barraged with choices when it comes to managing the symptoms of menopause and confronting the increased threat of disease associated with getting older. And my guess is that media attention and product marketing have escalated our fears about menopause in an effort to both educate us and, more important, sell us on medicines or herbal remedies. For decades, menopause—a term that simply means a woman's final menstrual period and the end of fertility—was pretty much a quiet, private affair. With all of the media attention menopause has received, it's hard to imagine that many women have little or no difficulty with this particular biological transition. (Indeed, in many cultures there is no word for hot flashes.) Today, there's continuous media banter about *perimenopausal symptoms* and *postmenopausal afflictions,* as though we're preparing ourselves for a major war with our bodies. A woman of "a certain age" may feel as though she has warning lights flashing from her ovaries. If you're peri-menopausal, the warning is, "Danger! Could overheat at any moment! Emotionally unstable. Keep a wide berth!" If you're postmenopausal, the message is "Warning! Wide Body (notice the weight gain?). Prone to Sudden Stops (heart attack), Blowouts (fractures from weakening bones), and Unpredictable Turns (a sign of Alzheimer's?)."

It's difficult to determine how many of the physical and emotional challenges we're experiencing are truly the result of menopause and our fluctuating and diminishing estrogen supply. Which of them are simply a matter of the general impact of growing older, or the result of our attitudes toward aging? Which are the effect of entering a time in our lives when stress and responsibility may be peaking?

The ten- to twenty-year span that covers the time before menopause begins through the time after it ends, when a woman is hormonally different from how she was before the changes started occurring and how she will be after her body "settles out," also happens to be a very emotionally compelling time. Our children may be rebelling or leaving home; our parents may be losing their health, their minds, or both. Our jobs may be demanding more of our time, energy, and creativity. And our marriages may be crumbling under the stress or fading into oblivion from lack of attention. Some of us may be facing up to our mortality for the first time, or with a new sense of urgency. Any of these life stresses could lead us to feel depressed, fatigued, anxious, disinterested in sex, or more prone to disease, with or without the hormonal fluctuations.

Modern medicine and the media seem to portray menopause less as a natural transition and more as a disease, a disease that *all* women will get, sooner or later. The mainstream treatment of choice for years was hormones—namely estrogen and progesterone, known as hormone replacement therapy (HRT). But recent research has revealed that there are risks, and serious ones, to HRT. Rather than protecting us from heart attacks, HRT may contribute to them. Rather than protecting us from cancer, it may lead to cancer. Rather than protecting us from Alzheimer's disease, HRT may be another risk factor. Estrogen, as far as we know, doesn't really stave off wrinkles or keep skin more supple. Are we certain to become victims of osteoporosis if we don't take estrogen? If we don't want to take estrogen, what else can we do to treat our symptoms and protect our health? This is not a book to help you determine whether or not you should take HRT for your hot flashes, night sweats, vaginal atrophy, bone loss, or other menopausal symptoms. That's for you and your health practitioner to decide. It's a complex question that depends greatly on the intensity of your symptoms, your personal health history, and your preferences.

First, let's sort out the actual symptoms associated with menopause and see where exercise will and won't help. Then we'll talk about how exercise can protect you from other health issues that can crop up as we age. Maybe you know you should exercise, but you don't know precisely why, or just how truly valuable exercise is. Or maybe when you read about the benefits of exercise in the past, heart attacks, strokes, or bone loss seemed part of a far too distant future to get you moving. Menopause may be just the impetus you need!

## Can Exercise Ease Your Menopausal Symptoms?

Let's review the symptoms and health concerns most women have with regard to menopause, and what they mean to your current and future health, and put them in perspective. While there are no guarantees that exercise will impact your particular menopausal symptom, you can conduct your own research using the chart provided at the end of this section.

**Hot flashes** are probably the number one reason women seek HRT during their menopausal years. But did you know that women who exercise regularly tend to report fewer menopausal symptoms that those who don't? Maybe women who exercise aren't bothered by sudden sweats and steamy faces as much as more sedentary women. Or maybe regular exercise boosts their moods or soothes their anxiety so much they forget to complain about or focus on their menopausal symptoms. At this point, nobody seems to know. So far, studies have not shown that adding exercise after hot flashes have started has any impact on their frequency or intensity. Still, yoga practitioners claim that forward bends (hanging the head lower than the heart) and inverted poses can help "cool" the body and reduce the intensity and frequency of hot flashes. (For more on these poses, see the yoga section on page 169.)

*Depression, moodiness, and sleep disturbances* can be related to hormonal changes, but they can also be associated with life changes and sleep deprivation. Regular exercise helps to boost mood, treat mild depression, enhance sleep and the ability to fall asleep, and improve cognitive function. One thing I do miss since menopause is falling asleep at night and waking up in the *morning*. But the problem is no longer night sweats—it's having to get up and go to the bathroom. That seems to be a fact of life. You can help yourself by monitoring your liquids after dinner. I've learned to keep a clear path between the bed and the bathroom—I can almost sleepwalk my way through it.

*Vaginal and urogenital complaints* such as itching, burning, infections, and painful intercourse can be a real problem. The vaginal walls do thin and the vagina actually shortens. Your doctor might suggest using herbal remedies and topical applications as alternatives to taking estrogen or using topical estrogen creams. Exercise is not considered effective treatment; however, exercise is linked to increased sex drive and feelings of self-esteem. Pelvic floor exercises, such as Kegels, can help with loss of bladder control. To isolate the muscles used when doing a Kegel, practice halting the flow of urine as you sit on the toilet. Once you've located the pelvic floor muscles, simply tighten and relax them at regular intervals throughout your day.

*Weight gain* is not known to be a result of menopause or lack of estrogen. Some women claim they lose weight on estrogen therapy, others claim they gain. Eating habits, a sedentary lifestyle, and the natural, progressive loss of muscle mass are the major conspirators that pack on pounds for most women. Aerobic exercise, resistance training, and overhauling your eating habits are your best bets for controlling weight gain. *But don't confuse thinness with health.* This is another area where the media may be going overboard. Because of the images we see in magazines, we tend to equate getting fitter with getting thin. But you can increase your fitness without losing weight. And studies show that exercise can still be very protective of your health and well-being regardless of your weight.

Does your **low sex drive** leave you wishing for a Viagra for women? Lack of sex drive after menopause may not be related to estrogen levels. Some postmenopausal women enjoy sex more when they know they can't get pregnant. On the other hand, if vaginal atrophy has made intercourse uncomfortable, that's certainly going to dampen your desire. Plus, you may be affected by such powerful sexual inhibitors as a heavy workload, daily stressors, a negative body image, or boredom or emotional resentments. Regular exercisers report better sex lives, perhaps because exercise helps reduce the effects of stress, promotes circulation throughout the body, including to the pelvic and genital areas, helps you relax, and generates self-esteem.

When I was working full-time and trying to help care for my mother, I thought my libido had dried up and blown away. But when I found time to relax and exercise, I realized that stress was sapping my energy and was the main cause of my low libido. I tried some suggested herbal and hormonal remedies to boost desire, but I still believe that exercise—the more vigorous the better—is my best and safest bet.

*Forgetfulness* is a haunting symptom of aging. Many of us fear the loss of our mental abilities as well as the onset of Alzheimer's disease. Stress, not hormones, is probably responsible for what some women call menopausal moments. Sometimes such forgetfulness is just a matter of too much on your plate, which keeps you from storing information properly. Exercise definitely reduces the physiological effects of stress and helps boost brainpower.

If you have concerns about Alzheimer's disease, I highly recommend reading the book *Aging with Grace: What the Nun Study Teaches Us about Leading Longer, Healthier, and More Meaningful Lives,* by David Snowdon, Ph.D. When my mother began suffering from memory problems, I took a personal crash course in Alzheimer's, reading books and online resources and talking to nurses and doctors who cared for my mom. Dr. Snowdon puts so much of the information I was struggling with into perspective. Rather than leaving us to grasp at snippets of research and news flashes on possibilities of new drug remedies, the Nun Study gives a complete overview of lifestyle habits and their potential to ward off this devastating disease. It is a complete story, a fascinating book written with wisdom and humor, and Dr.

Snowdon covers all the basics, from nature to nurture, from food and exercise to how learning may impact the brain. And after years of analyzing that data, what is Dr. Snowdon's primary recommendation? Walk.

**Bone loss** is driven by lack of estrogen, lack of exercise, and not enough calcium in the diet. The National Osteoporosis Foundation suggests the following preventive methods: First, get enough calcium and vitamin D. (Postmenopausal women need 1,500 milligrams of calcium a day. As for vitamin D, exposure to sunlight for ten to fifteen minutes a day on the skin of our faces, hands, and arms usually gives our bodies all that it needs. But as we age, we are less able to manufacture it. Windows, clothing, and pollution all affect how much vitamin D we get. So experts recommend taking between 400 and 800 IU of vitamin D a day in the form of a multivitamin. Natural sources of vitamin D include egg yolks, saltwater fish, and liver.) Second, get regular weight-bearing exercise, such as walking. (Women who are very small and thin may need to carry a weighted backpack when walking in order to stimulate bone growth.) Third, stop smoking and don't drink alcohol excessively. Fourth, talk to your doctor about bone health. Fifth, have a bone density test and take medication when appropriate. Getting tested is important because you can't make assumptions about bone health. My mother was quite thin and smoked as much as a pack of cigarettes a day. At eighty, she had her first bone density test. She looked like she had osteoporosis because her posture was so stooped from spending hours bending over a craft project or an easel. But the doctor said she had "the bones of a thirty year old." Go figure.

**Heart disease and stroke** become more of a risk for women after menopause because of changes in the blood and arteries. But aerobic exercise, including walking, can reverse these changes! Yes, even the flexibility and health of your arteries! Walking improves your cholesterol profile, though there is some controversy as to whether blood cholesterol levels are as important as we once thought. Today, researchers are examining the relationship between inflammation and heart disease. Now doctors are looking to inflammation markers, like the c-reactive protein test, to assess a patient's risk for heart disease. The Harvard Physicians' Health Study found that high levels of c-reactive protein proved to be an early warning sign for first heart attacks six to eight years later. Exercise will also help lower c-reactive protein.

## Beyond Menopause

In addition to the concerns listed above, aging brings health concerns unrelated to menopause, such as cancer, diabetes, and arthritis.

The American Cancer Society recommends exercising thirty minutes a day at least five days a week to help prevent *cancer*. Experts note that lifestyle behaviors, including what you eat and how much you exercise, are among the most important factors that determine your risk of getting the disease in some form. More than half a million deaths a year can be linked to unhealthy eating and lack of exercise. Breast cancer, ovarian cancer, and colorectal cancer seem to have the strongest exercise link so far—and exercising more vigorously and longer may have a more protective effect. Scientists are still searching for the reason why exercise is important; it's a complicated science teasing out all the data in these studies. But the link is definitely there. (For more information on the link between exercise and cancer, visit the American Cancer Society's Web site at www.cancer.org.)

*Diabetes* now affects more than eighteen million people, or 6 percent of the U.S. population, according to the American Diabetes Association (www.diabetes.org). The body's inability to produce enough insulin or to use it effectively to carry sugar from the blood to the cells can lead to all sorts of complications, including heart disease, stroke, kidney failure, foot and skin problems, and nerve damage. Sometimes, the problems of diabetes can be completely overcome by healthy eating and a regular exercise program. If you need to take insulin, you may be able to take less if you walk briskly every day, which may help to control blood sugar levels.

The term *arthritis* is used for many different types of diseases, including fibromyalgia and rheumatoid arthritis, which are not age related. But osteoarthritis is a disease of age that involves degenerative changes in our joints that create inflammation and lead to pain. It may affect only one joint or many. I have arthritis in my feet, knees, and neck. For many years, doctors thought that exercise was bad for people with arthritis. But today we know that exercise can help reduce pain, stiffness, and inflammation and support the joints by maintaining strong muscles. Plus, like other sedentary people, those with arthritis who don't exercise put themselves at risk for other diseases, such as heart disease, diabetes, and cancer. (If you have arthritis, you should check with your doctor about how to start an exercise program and whether you may need to pre-medicate before a walk or other exercise session.)

## Moving Beyond Midlife with Energy, Strength, and Grace

Menopause does mark a major transition in most women's lives. But it is a far more serious and creative transition than the hot flashes or night sweats that might accompany it. Many women come to this time in their lives in fear and transition out of it with confidence, a new sense of purpose, and a zest for living. Menopause definitely presses our mortality up against us. But in doing so, it makes us take stock of our lives and decide what's really important to us and what we can leave behind. Many of us are suddenly free to pursue our own dreams or recover lost parts of ourselves. We may finally have the time, resources, patience, and confidence to stop doing what's expected of us and start doing what we want to do.

Whether that's hiking the Alps in Switzerland, learning to play a musical instrument, tackling a new profession that's miles from the one we've been doing, starting a business, going back to school, playing with our grandkids, joining a local theater company, or renewing our marriages (or moving on), we're poised to transition into what may be the most creatively fertile and potent time of our lives.

And regular exercise, like walking, may be one of our safest, most reliable allies from this point forward.

### Your Personal Menopause Research

1. Make a list of the measurable menopausal symptoms bothering you most at this time, such as hot flashes, night sweats, tiredness, sleepless nights, moodiness, or feeling depressed. You may want to focus on just one symptom, or several. Fill in the ones you want to focus on under "symptom" in the chart. At the beginning or end of each day, check the box if you are experiencing or experienced that symptom. (For instance, in the morning, you might want to note that you woke up several times during the night, so check sleepless night. By evening you may forget! At the end of the day, you might mark how many hot flashes you had that day.)

2. At the same time you begin logging your symptoms into this chart, start your walking program. (Read "Beginner Basics" on page 25 first. You might want to start with the "Count Your Steps to a Healthier Future" program.)

3. After a month, review the frequency and intensity of your symptoms and evaluate whether exercise has had any impact.

|  | Symptom | Symptom | Symptom | Symptom | Walking/min |
|---|---|---|---|---|---|
|  |  |  |  |  |  |
| **Monday** |  |  |  |  |  |
|  |  |  |  |  |  |
| **Tuesday** |  |  |  |  |  |
|  |  |  |  |  |  |
| **Wednesday** |  |  |  |  |  |
|  |  |  |  |  |  |
| **Thursday** |  |  |  |  |  |
|  |  |  |  |  |  |
| **Friday** |  |  |  |  |  |
|  |  |  |  |  |  |
| **Saturday** |  |  |  |  |  |
|  |  |  |  |  |  |
| **Sunday** |  |  |  |  |  |
|  |  |  |  |  |  |
| **Totals** |  |  |  |  |  |

| | | Symptom | Symptom | Symptom | Symptom | Walking/min |
|---|---|---|---|---|---|---|
| | | | | | | |
| **Monday** | | | | | | |
| | | | | | | |
| **Tuesday** | | | | | | |
| | | | | | | |
| **Wednesday** | | | | | | |
| | | | | | | |
| **Thursday** | | | | | | |
| | | | | | | |
| **Friday** | | | | | | |
| | | | | | | |
| **Saturday** | | | | | | |
| | | | | | | |
| **Sunday** | | | | | | |
| | | | | | | |
| **Totals** | | | | | | |

|  | Symptom | Symptom | Symptom | Symptom | Walking/min |
|---|---|---|---|---|---|
|  |  |  |  |  |  |
| Monday |  |  |  |  |  |
|  |  |  |  |  |  |
| Tuesday |  |  |  |  |  |
|  |  |  |  |  |  |
| Wednesday |  |  |  |  |  |
|  |  |  |  |  |  |
| Thursday |  |  |  |  |  |
|  |  |  |  |  |  |
| Friday |  |  |  |  |  |
|  |  |  |  |  |  |
| Saturday |  |  |  |  |  |
|  |  |  |  |  |  |
| Sunday |  |  |  |  |  |
|  |  |  |  |  |  |
| **Totals** |  |  |  |  |  |

|  | Symptom | Symptom | Symptom | Symptom | Walking/min |
|---|---|---|---|---|---|
|  |  |  |  |  |  |
| Monday |  |  |  |  |  |
|  |  |  |  |  |  |
| Tuesday |  |  |  |  |  |
|  |  |  |  |  |  |
| Wednesday |  |  |  |  |  |
|  |  |  |  |  |  |
| Thursday |  |  |  |  |  |
|  |  |  |  |  |  |
| Friday |  |  |  |  |  |
|  |  |  |  |  |  |
| Saturday |  |  |  |  |  |
|  |  |  |  |  |  |
| Sunday |  |  |  |  |  |
|  |  |  |  |  |  |
| Totals |  |  |  |  |  |

# Chapter Two

# Walking for Life

*"There is no better time than the years surrounding menopause for a woman to start or renew an exercise program."*

—Physician and Sports Medicine, *July 1996*

Walking may well be the miracle "drug" of the twenty-first century, the near-perfect antidote to the sedentary lifestyle of the computer age. It's a "treatment" that can often serve as preventive medicine as well as a prescription for healing; a pill with no bitter taste or negative side effects, except soreness or blisters. If a manufacturer could package all the benefits of walking into a single pill, they'd make billions of dollars.

Walking comes with one major price tag: It takes time. Things that take a bite out of your day, day after day, require motivation. Motivation is a finicky thing. It can disappear like morning dew on a blade of grass when the sun rises. One day you're filled with excitement and energy as you look forward to your next walk, and the next day, you seem to totally forget the feelings that buoyed you to invest in a new pair of walking shoes and a book like this! Boredom can strangle motivation. Busyness can submerge it. Even talk of "discipline" can sabotage it. The kid in us rebels. Motivation comes more from the heart than the head. You have to keep feeding it the right fruits: knowledge, creativity, and variety.

Whether you're approaching menopause or past it, you can easily see the benefits of becoming active and staying active for the rest of your life. It all seems so obvious and simple, doesn't it? Our bodies were built to move, and when we move them enough every day, they stay healthier, we feel happier, and we are far more likely to live longer (and enjoy the extra years!). It's really a no-brainer, and yet we sit. We think about it, we stew about it, we make excuses about it. What we need to reap a healthier, happier future is far more about *inspiration* than perspiration. We don't have to work hard physically to reap the healthful rewards of exercise, but sometimes we have to work hard mentally and emotionally to overcome inertia. We need mental stamina and emotional energy to get off the couch or out from behind the desk or away from the TV. And that's where this book comes in. It's full of programs to inspire you to continue to get enough daily exercise for *the rest of your life*.

Some people don't seem to require a lot of variety in their exercise lives. They have the kind of personalities that love routine. Once they start a program, they stick with it, day after day. I had a friend at *Prevention* magazine who had been walked every day for fourteen years, barely skipping a day. She met friends, dogs in tow, and they walked several miles together, rain or shine, summer and winter. But lots of us are not that steady. We get bored easily. We get distracted from our exercise goals. We get busy, fall out of the habit, and then need to be inspired all over again.

I created the programs that follow to match a variety of moods and life circumstances you may find yourself in now or at some future date. For instance, you may be going through a very stressful time period, taking care of an aging parent or meeting a challenging deadline at work. Or perhaps you'd like to meditate regularly but can't find the time or can't sit still when you do. The "Stress Reduction" program may be just what you need to help melt away stress and ease anxiety.

Or you may be trying to take off some extra pounds or get more physically fit, and you're looking for a more dynamic walking program than what your usual routine provides. Preparing for a 5K race or using the "Power Up Plus" program could be just the ticket that excites you and provides the results you want. Perhaps you became glued to the couch during a particularly harsh winter and now you need the inspiration and spiritual enrichment that can be gained by walking in beautiful natural surroundings. The "Nature and Gardens for Healing and Rejuvenation" program could give you a whole new perspective on the flow of life and the power of plants and nature to support and nourish our spirits.

Or maybe you're a grandmother (or a late-blooming mom), and you'd like to involve children or grandchildren in your active lifestyle. The "Hang with Your Grandchildren" walking program will give you some creative ideas for passing on the exercise lifestyle to future generations.

One thing is for certain: Keeping track of your efforts will help you get started and stay the course. Research has shown that people who write things down are more likely to follow through on them. Keeping records and logs helps us to stay on track, see results, and solidify our intentions. This book can serve as your workbook and log—a place where you can plot your course and mark your progress. Keep it handy, perhaps right by your bed or breakfast table. May it become well worn around the edges as you use it!

## Beginner Basics

First, we're going to focus on the basics for beginners. How far, how fast, how long should you walk? How do you get started? For some, it can be as easy as slipping on a pair of comfortable shoes and heading out the door. But many of us need a plan and some parameters.

First of all, if you have any kind of existing health condition, if you're taking medications on a regular basis, and especially if you have heart disease or diabetes, check with your doctor before you begin a walking program. Walking is usually safe for everyone, but if you have specific health problems, you may need specialized recommendations from your health care provider. It's important that you let your doctor know about any change in your daily routine. Getting more exercise can sometimes reduce the need for certain medications, and your doctor may want to see you more often to help regulate dosages. One thing is for sure: Your doctor should be thrilled that you want to exercise more and happy to help you in any way. If your doctor isn't helpful, maybe it's time for a switch. Look for a doctor who can be an inspiration and set a good example for you.

If you're healthy as far as you know, walking is the best and safest way to start becoming more active. Just be aware that chest pain, heart palpitations, dizziness, nausea, headaches, or leg pain brought on by exercise require a follow-up with your doctor.

Second, if you have problems with your feet that cause discomfort on a regular basis, see an orthopedist or podiatrist for recommendations on treatment and footwear. Your feet are your primary walking tools. If they give you trouble, you're just not going to walk. (But you can always swim or even bike, so don't let painful feet stop you from getting a healthy dose of activity in your life.) Corns, bunions, hammertoes, and the like can be a painful annoyance. People with diabetes need to be especially careful to choose socks and shoes that fit properly and don't rub or chafe. Some foot pain can be controlled or eased by proper footwear. Over-the-counter inserts and orthotics can help, too. Invest in your feet—they're worth it!

## 30 Minutes a Day

In July of 1996, the surgeon general of the United States released *The Report on Physical Activity and Health,* which basically proclaimed inactivity as hazardous to your health. The report reviewed three decades of research on physical activity, amassing enough information to place physical activity in the limelight as a cornerstone to healthy living. The report was unequivocal: It asserted that not exercising was as dangerous as smoking in terms of dire health consequences. It was a landmark report and a momentous occasion for everyone involved in health care, health promotion, and the sports or exercise industry. And it was definitive for all of us in terms of how much we needed to be active, recommending "a moderate amount of physical activity most, if not all, days of the week." What's a moderate amount? Activity that burns 150 extra calories a day, or 1,000 calories a week. That translates into walking 1 3/4 miles at a twenty-minute-per-mile pace (thirty minutes of walking) or walking two miles in thirty minutes (a fifteen-minute-per-mile pace). To reach the minimum goal, you could also walk up stairs or jump rope or run at a ten-minute-per-mile pace for fifteen minutes. More exercise tends to confer more health and fitness benefits. But the people who have the most to gain healthwise from physical activity are those who move from the couch to the sidewalk.

Further research confirmed that you didn't even have to walk that mile and three-quarters all at once. Three ten-minute bouts of brisk walking will give you the same health benefits as thirty minutes all at once. It will also burn about the same amount of calories.

If you've been sedentary, meaning you've not done much more than walk from your couch to the dinner table or from your bed to the car, and you sit all day long at your work, then you'll want to start slowly, with short bursts of walking—just five- or ten-minute strides several times a day. For greater fitness and endurance, you'll want to work up to walking thirty minutes or more all at once. But when you're crunched for time, shorter walks are better than none at all.

How fast do you need to walk to reap the benefits? A comfortably brisk pace will do. That will be a different speed for different people, depending on your age, your fitness level, your weight, and other factors. So I'm not going to tell you to walk a twenty-minute or a fifteen-minute mile, which would require that you measure your course and time yourself, or tell you to find your target heart rate and take your pulse. Instead, all you need to know is that you should walk as fast as feels comfortable, yet you should still be able to carry on a conversation—no gasping for breath. A good way to think of it is that you are walking with a purpose. Imagine you're walking to get to a meeting or catch a train, and you're just a little bit late. A casual stroll is fine for right after a meal, when you don't want to tax your digestive system. But your thirty-minute walk should be comfortably brisk. Keep in mind that you want to feel energized and relaxed when you're finished, not pooped!

## Beginner Tools

I've already mentioned that research shows that writing down your daily activity helps people stay active, so this book or a calendar or logbook is an important tool for success. Probably most important are a good pair of shoes and socks. You can walk in just about any kind of clothing; unless it's very hot or you are very overweight, you probably won't sweat much when walking a mile in twenty minutes. That makes it especially easy to take a walk during work hours. There's no real need to change your clothes, except to slip on a pair of walking shoes and socks.

That's not to say that walking can't be a great excuse to buy new clothes. Having a favorite pair of sweats, a luxuriously soft and perspiration-wicking T-shirt, or a colorful windbreaker to grab when you're going for a walk adds pleasure to your routine. If you'll be walking outside during frigid winter temperatures, then of course you'll have to invest in layers of outdoor gear to keep comfortable from head to foot.

For some women, a sports bra is a workout essential. If your breasts bounce when you're striding, you'll be uncomfortable and perhaps even self-conscious. Sports bras are widely available these days in all varieties of style and support. I like the one-piece variety that doesn't have any hooks to press into your flesh, even if I do get completely tangled up in them sometimes when I try to put them on.

## Picking Your Walking Shoes

There are a myriad of fitness shoes on the market that will work for walking. The best choice for you depends on your foot, the climate, the terrain you'll be walking on, and your budget. Go for the best you can afford. Remember, you're protecting a very important asset with those dollars.

I'm a sales shopper. Rarely do I buy a pair of walking shoes at full price. So while most of the best brands run in the $60 to $90 range, I often pay much less. I'll also take advantage of online sales, as long as I'm familiar with the brand name and know how the shoes fit my foot.

While writing for *Prevention* magazine, I primarily recommended walking shoes, because it seemed to make sense that shoes designed specifically for walking would serve people best. But recently I've talked with many people who prefer running shoes, especially racewalkers, because of their increased cushioning and flexibility. Because of a particular problem with my feet, an orthopedist once suggested I wear running shoes for more protection. So I suggest you experiment to find what works best for you. Below are just a few points to keep in mind when shoe shopping:

- Shop at the end of the day, when your feet are at their largest.

- Wear or bring your favorite pair of socks with you. Or buy a pair at the store.

- Trace the outline of your feet onto a piece of paper or cardboard, cut it out, and bring it with you to the store. If that pattern doesn't fit on the bottom of a shoe you're trying on, don't buy it. Workout shoes can be deceptively comfortable when you first put them on but hurt later when you're walking in them, usually because you've bought them too small.

- When standing in the shoe, press down beyond your longest toe (or have someone do it for you). There should be about a finger's width of space between your longest toe (not necessarily your big toe) and the end of the shoe. Your feet need some room to move inside the shoe and to expand as you walk. I see so many people who wear athletic shoes with their big or middle toes poking out over the front of the shoe.

- Fit the largest foot first. (One foot is almost always slightly bigger than the other.)

- If you wear any type of orthotic or padding, make sure that fits in the shoe comfortably.

- Take the time to walk around in the shoes, preferably on a hard surface. If you're at the mall and the store is carpeted, ask if you can walk up and down the linoleum outside the store to see how the shoe feels. After all, most of your walking will be done on a hard surface rather than a soft, yielding surface.

I have always liked New Balance shoes. In fact, they are the only company I know of that produces a racewalking shoe that is really flexible enough to support that kind of walking. Right now I have several pairs, one for racewalking, some with sturdier soles, and even a pair with Velcro instead of laces. (On some days when my back is sore, I hate to have to bend over and tie my shoes while I'm out for a walk!) New Balance is one of the few brands that come in a variety of widths, too. And I need a wide shoe. Other good brands include Saucony, Adidas, Ryka, Avia, Brooks, and Easy Spirit. I also have some light hikers that I use for dirt roads and easy hiking trails and for walking in sloppy winter weather. They can be a bit more expensive, but they really last and are invaluable on rugged terrain. My collection includes Merrells, New Balance, Timberland, Vasque, and Mephisto.

And finally, I have a pair of Teva walking sandals. I've always been amazed at how well they fit, how comfortable they are, and what great traction they have. On hot summer days, they are really great. Besides, they give you a chance to get rid of sock-line tans.

## Anytime Is a Good Time

Over the years, many people have asked me when the best time is to walk. I've always said, "Whatever time is most convenient is the best time." Some research seems to show that there may be some advantage to walking before breakfast if you're trying to burn fat, but if you're not an early bird and you keep missing those walks, then you're not burning much fat.

Walking is a great energizer. If you can manage it, a late-afternoon walk during a break or on the way home from work can be just the pick-me-up you need to face kitchen duty or to wake up for a movie or evening entertainment. Our tendency is to grab coffee or a sugary snack, but a brisk walk will be so much more effective. If you have trouble sleeping or falling asleep, walking can be a great asset, but some people get a little too wide awake if they walk after dinner.

I'm a morning walker myself. For one thing, it just fits well with my schedule and my constitution. I'm up with the sun, usually, which means 5:30 or 6:00 in the summer and around 7:00 in the winter. And I love the freshness of the air, the glisten of morning dew on the grass, and the sounds of chirping birds. In the summer, it's simply the best way to beat the heat. For me, it works. Then I'll sometimes walk again, later in the day, after sitting at the computer for too many hours. But that walk is usually more leisurely. It's more an effort to stretch my limbs and clear my mind than to get a workout. I often walked during my lunch hour, especially in the winter months. Partners were usually plentiful, and we'd often walk first and then grab a bite to eat.

I would love to walk more at night, but the country roads where I live are just not safe and we have no sidewalks. But I fondly remember walking home in the dark when I was a teen growing up in Westfield, New Jersey. I just love walking by houses that are all lit up and allow you to get a glimpse of the life they carry on the inside. Our house, was always lit from top to bottom—a very welcoming and cheery sight! There's something wonderfully mysterious and otherworldly about walking after dark. But of course, safety is sometimes a concern. A group of people in Bethlehem, Pennsylvania, which is near where I live, started a night walking group, called the Moonwalkers, that met several nights a week for years after dinner was over and the kids were in bed. They were mostly busy moms who felt this was the only time available to them for exercise. They didn't feel safe walking alone, but in a group they were fine.

## The Power of Partners

Finding someone to walk with on a regular basis is an absolute blessing for anyone who is trying to become more consistent in her efforts to get regular exercise. Most of us find it easier to keep a commitment to someone else than to ourselves when we're lying in bed on a cold morning, wondering if we should slip on our walking shoes or roll over for another fifteen minutes of sleep. Knowing that a friend is going to be waiting for us on a street corner is a foolproof motivator for most people. I think it's even better than a group, because then you can't say, "Well, someone will be there. They won't miss me."

Finding a partner seems to be something that occurs naturally or by serendipity. You just have to let people know that you're walking and you'd love to have company. Sooner or later, someone at work or in your neighborhood will turn up. Maybe they'll see you out there day after day and ask if they can join you. Or you can post a notice at church, the office, or your community center. (I think it would be great if doctors' and dentists' offices had bulletin boards for walkers to find buddies.)

You may find it most convenient to walk with the same person all the time. It is important that he or she has the same ability and pace as you. If you're walking fifteen-minute miles, you're going to feel cheated if you have to slow down to a twenty-minute-per-mile pace. And if your partner is pooped after a mile but you're ready for three more, that's not going to be very helpful. Personally, I like having different walking partners. Right now, I have a neighbor who is an early bird like me, likes to walk with poles, and matches my pace and distance. When I walk with her, I always stay out there longer than I would have alone. And she pushes my pace, too. I also enjoy making walking dates with friends and family members when our schedules allow it.

And, of course, there's always the dog. I'd never recommend anyone get a dog just to have a walking partner, but maybe you have a dog already that has never been walked regularly. He or she will benefit as much as you will from daily exercise! If you've been considering getting a dog for a variety of reasons, make sure you choose a breed that would love to walk with you and not be too much to handle. Dogs can be a great source of fun and joy on a walk. And they're never too tired or too busy when you want to head out the door. I love walking with medium- or small-sized dogs like my cockapoo or my son's Welsh corgis. Larger dogs can be good walking partners, but often big breeds like labs and golden retrievers really need to be run, and unless they are well trained, they'll end up dragging you down the street.

If you've found a walking partner, you've found a treasure. Treat him or her with respect. Be on time and keep your commitment. Call when you can't make it. Consider giving him or her a special gift during the holidays. Walking partners may not be your best friends or even people you spend time with other than on walks. But they are very important allies in your exercise program. Let them know how much you value their company!

To make it easy to do this, I have six different e-mail cards for walkers on my Web site, www.walkforallseasons.com. You participate in the design and add your own notes. They are a great way to say thanks or to set up a walking date. They're free and they're fun!

## Walking Technique

There are no special techniques you need to learn for basic, everyday walking. (If you want to use specialized fitness walking or racewalking technique, see the "Power Up Your Stride" program on page 67.) You've been walking around for close to half a century or more. So for the most part, you can just keep up the good work. However, many of us have developed poor postural habits over the years. Some bad habits we may have adopted during adolescence, when we stooped to hide our breasts or to be the same height as our slower-growing boyfriends! Many women I've observed have rounded shoulders and sunken chests, which only worsen with age. While our mothers may have told us to stand up straight when we were kids, it never seemed that important. But a comfortably straight posture with a lifted chest and head in alignment with our shoulders looks youthful and helps prevent aches and pains.

It takes a lot of conscious awareness to maintain good posture throughout your day. And when you first start rearranging your bones and muscles in an effort to stand taller and with better alignment, you'll probably feel worse! You need to stretch out certain muscles that have become too tight, and strengthen muscles that have become overstretched. Yoga poses can be very helpful for maintaining a supple, flexible back and improving posture. For that reason, I've included a whole section in the back of this book of my favorites. I became interested in yoga in my twenties but didn't practice it consistently until my forties, when my flexibility began to diminish and I suffered from bouts of lower-back pain. When I was fifty, I took 200 hours of hatha yoga teacher training and became a Registered Yoga Teacher (RYT). I find yoga to be the perfect complement to a daily walking program. Not only can yoga stretch and strengthen your body, it can calm your mind and help your concentration and focus.

Recently I developed neck pain, probably from too many hours spent slouching over a computer for the last twenty years combined with a whiplash injury. I researched yoga poses to help stretch and strengthen my neck and shoulders as well as open my upper chest and strengthen my upper back. Too often, when I sit in front of the computer, I let my head jut forward. Now that I've actually experienced pain as the result of years of neglect, I can finally remember to check my posture throughout the day as I type!

Every time you walk, you can work on your posture. You want to stand tall, with your head aligned over your shoulders, shoulders over hips, hips over ankles. Your shoulders should be relaxed. Don't force them back in military posture. Lift your chest so that you're not resting your rib cage on your diaphragm, which is what happens whenever you slouch forward. It's a slight movement that makes a world of difference in how you look and feel. To experiment, stand in your normal, relaxed posture and place your fingertips on your breastbone. Push forward and upward against your fingertips, and notice the shift in your rib cage and your ability to breathe easier.

While some walking coaches advise tucking your buttocks under and pulling in your stomach, I've never been able to walk that way. But it's important to bring your pelvis into proper alignment. The image I learned from Dynamic Walking founder Suki Munsell, Ph.D., is much more helpful. Dr. Munsell suggested pressing your belly button toward your backbone as you walk. This helps strengthen core muscles and helps drop the pelvis into proper position. Stand and try this right now. With your knees soft, not locked, stand tall and press your navel back toward your spine and notice the shift as your tailbone drops toward the ground. You don't need to squeeze hard or tightly, just enough to adjust your posture. If you practice it often enough, it may begin to become second nature, though I still check myself. I tend to stand and walk with a swayback, which compresses the lower back and can lead to pain, even sciatica. Standing tall, with proper alignment, has definitely helped me.

Let your arms swing naturally as you walk. But don't throw your energy away by letting them flap and fidget every which way. (Once you become conscious of this, you'll notice people who walk like scarecrows, with arms flapping in the breeze.) Cup your hands slightly and keep your arms swinging like pendulums, forward and back in a straight line. If you notice that one arm seems to swing harder than the other, try to balance out your arm swing left to right, to avoid unnecessary twisting of your torso.

Don't drop your head and stare at your feet when you walk. That puts tremendous strain on your neck and may even contribute to feelings of depression. Your feet will avoid pitfalls in your path if you just scan the area in front of you. If you're dropping your head to avoid bright sun, get some sunglasses and wear a visor to cut the glare. You'll be much more comfortable!

## Stretches for Walkers

You should use several basic stretches with any of the walking programs in this book. In addition to these basic stretches, you will find a special section on page 169 that details useful yoga postures. Because these postures help stretch and strengthen the body, I've found them to be particularly helpful to my walking program.

Always stretch after you have warmed up for a few minutes by walking. You'll get much more out of the stretch when you've gotten your muscles a little warmed up than if you try to stretch cold. Stretch again at the end of your session. Tight calf muscles can lead to plantar fasciitis, which is an inflammation of tissue on the bottom of the foot. Most people refer to the condition as heel pain or heel spurs. Regular stretching and gradual conditioning can help avoid it, which is preferable, since it can be difficult to reverse once you have it! Tight hamstrings can contribute to lower-back pain. All in all, stretching protects you from injury and feels great, so take some time to do it.

# Count Your Steps to a Healthier Future

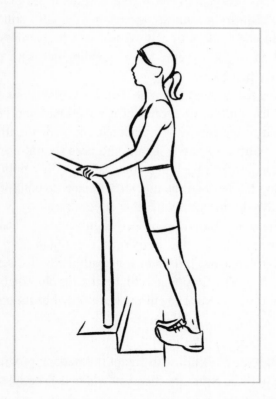

**Calves:** Stand on a step or curb with your heel hanging over the edge. You may need a pole or wall for balance. Balancing on your toes, let your heel drop down till you feel a nice stretch in the calf muscle. This stretch seems to work better and more consistently than simply stretching one leg out behind and dropping the heel into the ground.

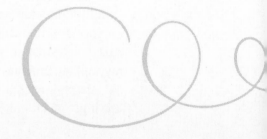

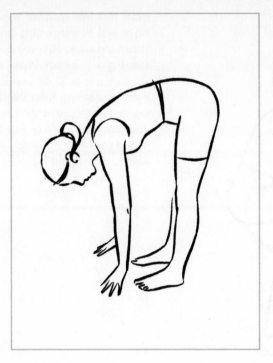

**Hamstrings:** Simple forward bends help stretch the backs of your legs. Just go slowly, rolling down, chin to chest, one vertebra at a time. If your back hurts and you can't let your arms dangle in front, rest your hands on your thighs for support. Breathe deeply as you relax into the stretch. Or, if there is a bench or steps nearby, you can lift your heel onto the bench, balancing on one leg, and fold forward over the extended leg until you feel a nice stretch. Don't bounce or force yourself to go lower than is comfortable.

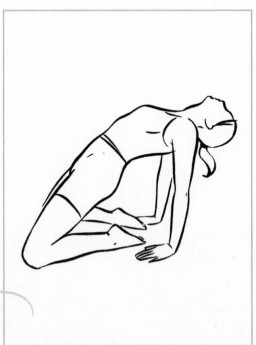

**Quadriceps:** Walkers don't seem to need to stretch the front of the thigh as much as other parts of the leg, unless you're training really hard or doing a lot of hills. One common way to stretch this muscle is to swing one leg back and catch it with your hand, behind your buttocks. But this can be hard for a lot of people to do. I like simply kneeling on the floor, then sitting back on my haunches and placing my hands on the floor behind my buttocks. If you then press your knees toward the ground, you'll feel a nice stretch.

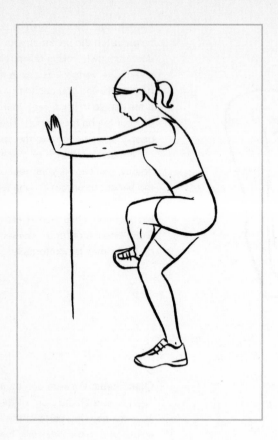

**Hips:** Your hips get tight from walking as well as from sitting too much. Here's a great stretch you can do standing or in a chair. Place one foot across the knee of the opposite leg. If you're standing, bend the standing leg, as though you're about to sit. You may need a tree or pole for support. If you're sitting, simply lean forward, over the bent leg.

# The Programs

## Count Your Steps to a Healthier Future

**Use this program if you**
- have been very sedentary and really need to ease into an active lifestyle;
- have been exercising pretty regularly, but spend most of the day sitting once you slip off your sneakers;
- would love to have constant feedback to help you monitor your daily exercise goals;
- cannot imagine walking for thirty or more minutes at a time, but can see yourself becoming more active all day long;
- are already walking thirty to sixty minutes a day and aren't losing weight yet.

**What You'll Need:** An accurate step counter and a place to log your steps. (We've got that right here!)

*P*art of the problem with modern living is not just that we don't exercise with a capital E. Many of us don't move much at all anymore. While we feel like we're very busy all day long, most of our activity is mental, not physical. We talk on the phone, type at computers, ride in cars, sit at desks, watch TV. Washing machines and dryers, dishwashers, cars, riding mowers, leaf blowers, snow blowers, even robotic vacuum cleaners deprive our bodies of calorie-burning movement. Supermarkets and department stores keep us from walking downtown (if there is a downtown!). Fast food and pizza delivery keep us from expending calories in food preparation and cleanup. Sometimes our lack of activity is a matter of lifestyle changes that occur as we get older. Kids grow up, neighborhood and working conditions alter, or friends move away and we give up certain sports or activities we once enjoyed together.

In short, even when we *do* walk briskly for thirty minutes a day, our overall activity level throughout the day may be so compromised that we're still not burning enough calories to fight off weight gain or to lose weight.

As a single mom for ten years, I had cared for two growing boys, my own house, and a dog while working full-time. I lived in a townhouse that had a flight of stairs between every room. Laundry was in the basement, and my bedroom was on the third floor. My sons' rooms were on the fourth floor. I did all the cleaning myself, walked the dog, did all the laundry, folded it and put it away, and washed dishes by hand. When the boys fell asleep in the car, I carried them to their beds. I walked with my kids to school while they were young. When they got older, I walked to their sports games a few blocks away. I mowed my own little lawn and weeded my small garden. This was in addition to intentional exercise programs of walking for thirty or more minutes in the morning or at lunch, attending some aerobics classes, weight training, and recreational activities like biking, volleyball, tennis, and dancing.

When I turned forty, I remarried. I continued to exercise regularly, but the pounds piled on. In addition to aging and hormonal changes, my daily level of activity dramatically decreased. For instance, I moved into my husband's ranch-style home, with no stairs. The family dog was kept outside in a pen, so he no longer required walking three times a day. We lived in a rural area, too far from stores or schools to walk for shopping or sports events. I began commuting an hour a day instead of just twenty minutes, so I felt more pressed for time to exercise. We now had a dishwasher, plus a cleaning lady came twice a month. My husband took care of the lawn and the laundry. I had moved thirty minutes away from many of my walking buddies and active friends. That overall decrease in activity contributed to significant weight gain.

According to one source, sedentary American women walk between 2,000 and 7,000 steps a day. (My average, when I did not take an intentional exercise walk, was about 3,000 steps a day) When we were kids, we probably walked more like 10,000 to 14,000 steps a day. No wonder we can't eat the way we used to!

A Japanese public health promotion that centered on the idea of wearing a pedometer and walking 10,000 steps a day became very popular in 1964, when the Olympics were held in Tokyo and the benefits of exercise caught the public eye. The trend made its way to America in the late 1990s. By 2003, even McDonald's was handing out step counters to build a healthier public image.

Step counters can help you increase your activity level all day long, not just during a predetermined exercise period. Here's how to use them, whether you've been a couch potato for years and you want to ease yourself into an active lifestyle or you've been walking regularly but not losing weight:

Step counters range in price from $10 to $25. To determine if the one you're considering buying is good quality, put it on in the store and walk twenty steps. If it registers twenty, you've probably found a decent one. If it doesn't, look elsewhere.

Every morning as soon as you get out of bed, attach the step counter to your waistband, directly over your left or right hip bone. (If you don't have a waistband because you wear a dress, you can clip it to your underwear or pantyhose, but this isn't as effective because you can't check it periodically during the day.) Keep it on all day, and just before you go to bed, write down the number of steps you've taken. Reset it to zero.

The next morning, repeat. Do this for a week. Keep a daily log of the general kinds of activities you did. For instance, if you went shopping, write that down. If you spent most of the day traveling, record that. You're trying to get an idea of how your time is spent and how active or sedentary your day is and why.

Total up your number of steps for the week and divide by seven for an average daily step count. Or, if you have certain days when you are always more active, calculate separate step counts for your more active and less active days.

## Set Goals

Now that you have an idea of how many steps you normally take on any given day, set goals to increase them. It's best to increase gradually, so you don't get overwhelmed. For instance, you may decide you can add an extra 500 steps every day. Continue to wear the pedometer daily, and record your steps at the end of every day, logging the kinds of activities you did to increase your steps. Every kind of activity counts, from walking around while you talk on your cell phone to parking your car a few blocks away from your destination (or at the farthest end of the parking lot). You'll be surprised at how creative you can get when you have this constant tally going on. These little walking buddies are surprisingly motivational!

If you've been sedentary, continue to add steps to your day every week, until you reach a point where you don't feel like you can add many more steps to your day without doing some intentional exercise. By now, you may be feeling more energetic and enthusiastic about a walking program—and when you go for your first brisk ten-minute walk and see those steps pile up, you'll be a convert!

Begin by adding moderately brisk walks of eight to ten minutes several times a day. After all, that fits the surgeon general's recommendations for better health and protection from many life-threatening diseases: thirty minutes of brisk activity, like walking three to four miles per hour, most days of the week. Studies have shown that splitting that up into three shorter bouts works too. But just walking around all day, at a leisurely pace, no matter how many steps, is not the same thing. While more movement is better than none, we all know people who have jobs that keep them on their feet but who are anything but fit and healthy.

Eventually, you may want to graduate to a brisk thirty-minute or longer walk, most days of the week. In addition to all of the health benefits accrued through this level of exercise, you will also have more energy and vitality because of your increased endurance and higher intensity of exercise.

At this point, you may want to forget the pedometer. You're exercising regularly, so who needs it? Well, *I do*. If you want to *lose weight*, and your daily walk isn't doing it, you may want to continue watching your step counter, trying to get more bouts of activity or exercise or recreation into your day, until you see the scale begin a downward turn.

At *Prevention* magazine, we offered step counters to people who said they walked regularly but couldn't seem to lose weight, a common complaint. We told them to keep adding steps to their daily average until they started seeing some results. Most of these folks were walking 15,000 to 17,000 steps a day (about seven to eight-and-a-half miles) before the pounds started to drop. Their total number of steps included plenty of extra "lifestyle" steps, because they became more aware of how much sitting they normally did. But it also included some daily doses of continuous walking, as much as five to six miles a day, though this was sometimes spread over two walking periods. Many walked first thing in the morning and then just before or after dinner.

Some decided they'd better get more serious about curbing their appetites, because 17,000 steps a day was more than they felt they could maintain for a lifetime.

Overall, the step counter greatly increases your awareness of how active or inactive you are on any given day. It's up to you how much more active you want to become and in what way. Maybe you do love getting up during

TV commercials to do a little dancing or stepping in place. Or maybe you'd rather take a couple of brisk walks. It's up to you!

Don't underestimate the power of this little pedometer. Health promotion groups around the country report that their clients are finding it truly irresistible. If you don't have the resources of Hollywood stars, whose personal trainers practically move in with them, the step counter may be your personal electronic substitute. And it doesn't care what you look like at 6:00 A.M.

Here are some essential tips for the step-counting lifestyle:

- You may want to purchase a special clip, or create your own version, so that if the pedometer works its way off your waistband, it doesn't fall and break when it hits the ground.

- Be careful when heading to the bathroom. Thousands of pedometers have taking a dive into that bowl. Avoid fishing expeditions by removing it first or having a safety clip.

- Share your pedometer plan with friends. You may find an instant support group forming at work or at home. Chatting about all of the ways others get more steps in their day can help you find creative solutions.

- If you drive a lot, especially in a truck or vehicle that bounces around, leave your step counter open, or take it off in the car. It may register while you're sitting!

- Make sure that you can hear the device "clicking" as you walk. If it isn't making a sound, try moving it around a little bit till you know it's working properly.

- Use the log below to track your steps for one month—and general information on how you achieved them. Writing it down will help you focus, give you ideas for other days, and help you celebrate your progress. After thirty days, you can decide if you need to continue logging, or if you've developed the habits you need to support yourself without making daily notes. Return to step counting any time you feel the need to get back on track or boost your activity level.

# The 8-Week Step-Counting Program

## Week 1: Getting Your Baseline

Average number of steps per day: _____

| | Steps | Notes |
|---|---|---|
| **Monday** | | |
| | | |
| **Tuesday** | | |
| | | |
| **Wednesday** | | |
| | | |
| **Thursday** | | |
| | | |
| **Friday** | | |
| | | |
| **Saturday** | | |
| | | |
| **Sunday** | | |
| | | |
| **Totals** | | |

# Week 2: Goal: Add _____ steps per day.

Daily Goal: _____

| | Steps | Notes |
|---|---|---|
| **Monday** | | |
| | | |
| **Tuesday** | | |
| | | |
| **Wednesday** | | |
| | | |
| **Thursday** | | |
| | | |
| **Friday** | | |
| | | |
| **Saturday** | | |
| | | |
| **Sunday** | | |
| | | |
| **Totals** | | |

# Week 3: Goal: Add _____ steps per day.

Daily Goal: _____

| | Steps | Notes |
|---|---|---|
| **Monday** | | |
| | | |
| **Tuesday** | | |
| | | |
| **Wednesday** | | |
| | | |
| **Thursday** | | |
| | | |
| **Friday** | | |
| | | |
| **Saturday** | | |
| | | |
| **Sunday** | | |
| | | |
| **Totals** | | |

**Week 4: Goal: Add _____ steps per day.**

Daily Goal: _____

| | Steps | Notes |
|---|---|---|
| **Monday** | | |
| | | |
| **Tuesday** | | |
| | | |
| **Wednesday** | | |
| | | |
| **Thursday** | | |
| | | |
| **Friday** | | |
| | | |
| **Saturday** | | |
| | | |
| **Sunday** | | |
| | | |
| **Totals** | | |

# Foot Power: Walking as Transportation

**Try this program if you**
• are bored with walking in circles to get your exercise;
• are starting to feel silly driving to the health club to walk on the treadmill;
• live in an area where many places you frequent by car are actually within walking distance;
• want to feel connected to your neighborhood, meet people, and slow the pace of your life;
• have moved to a new, walkable neighborhood and are ready to scout the terrain;
• love multitasking, such as getting exercise while you take care of errands.

**What You'll Need:** A map of your town or city; appropriate comfortable shoes; weather-ready gear appropriate for your climate; a comfortable backpack, shopping bag, or personal shopping cart; knowledge of your comfortable walking pace for a mile.

*"Everything is within walking distance, if you have the time."*

—*Steven Wright, comedian*

Steven Wright's quote is plastered on my refrigerator. I laughed the first time I read it. But I also pondered the fact that people's idea of what is in walking distance has shrunk steadily over the last century. We think we don't have the time. *But is that really true?*

I grew up in the very walkable town of Westfield, New Jersey, where just about everyone could walk to church, synagogue, school, and shops, if they really wanted to, though few did. Some people walked to the train station in the center of town to commute to New York City. And we didn't have a mall nearby in those days (and still don't), so people did walk around downtown, once they found a parking spot. I walked to elementary school in the morning and even walked home for lunch, about five blocks each way. Junior high was about a mile away and the high school about a mile and a half.

When I got my driver's license at seventeen, I pretty much forgot that I had ever walked *anywhere*. I was the last child at home, so my mom let me use her car pretty much whenever I wanted to. I drove to school, to friends' houses, and to my after-school jobs. Driving was cool. Walking was not. What a concept!

When I became the walking editor at *Prevention* magazine at the age of thirty-four and started deliberately leaving my car behind and walking places that seemed within a reasonable distance, I remember this odd feeling coming over me, sort of a sense of déjà vu. I seemed to be triggering some unconscious memories of walking as a child. I realized I often felt a strong urge to cut through people's yards to get where I was going! As kids, we did that all the time. We had free access to everyone's backyards! As an adult, I was, thankfully, fully aware that cutting through someone's property could get me arrested, and maybe even shot at, so of course I disregarded that old familiar tug to take shortcuts! I remember feeling a little sad to realize I no longer had that freedom. But that feeling also made me very aware of just how long it had been since I'd relied on foot power to get around town!

At that point, my sisters had both lived most of their adult lives in New York City. When they heard that I'd become the first official "walking editor" for a national magazine, and that my job was to write a monthly column about walking for health and fitness, they didn't get it. Neither of them even *owned* a car at the time. They walked everywhere. In fact, I was so out of shape from driving *everywhere* that when I visited them in the city, I'd be hard-pressed to keep up with their pace!

The more I researched the benefits of exercise for my writing, the more I relied on walking as my preferred form of transportation whenever feasible. I walked all my lunch-time errands to the post office, the hairdresser, the pharmacy, or the bank. I met friends at downtown lunch spots. After work, I walked my sons to baseball practice, the grocery store, the pizza parlor, and the library. I found I really enjoyed walking with a purpose, just like I enjoyed walking to school as a kid. You get to see so much more on foot than you do from the behind the driver's seat! And you have more opportunity to interact with others, even if it's only a nod from a neighbor or a chance to lean down and pet somebody's dog. You feel connection—something often missing from our harried, automobile-dependent worlds.

When I moved to my current home in Williams Township, Pennsylvania—a house my husband built in the rural area where he grew up, I sorely missed the opportunity to walk around town. Now I live four miles from the nearest store, school, or post office, which isn't all that far, but the walk into town is down several long, steep hills, there are no sidewalks, and cars and trucks fly by at fifty miles per hour on country roads. While four miles on easy terrain might take me an hour, walking to town and back from here might take two, and I'd be a risk most of the way because of the lack of sidewalks.

But many of you are far more fortunate. The 1990 National Personal Transportation Study determined that 25 percent of all travel trips made by car are *one mile or less*! Forty percent are two miles or less. Almost half are three miles or less. Plus 53 percent of everyone in this country lives less than two miles from a bus or train station, making a walk-transit commute a convenient possibility.

You may be lucky enough to live and work in areas where walking could be a real transportation option for you. The use of your car may simply be a convenient habit and something you've never thought about changing. But now, as you consider the health benefits of walking, you may find a variety of ways and times to leave your car at home, or at least park a mile or so from your destinations and get your exercise while doing errands, shopping, or going to work or "play."

Not only will you be helping yourself to better health, you'll be improving the health of your community. First of all, you're reducing air pollution and conserving natural resources by driving your car less. And second, studies have shown that when people walk in an area, it becomes safer. Walkers notice things that are out of the ordinary—suspicious people or actions, mail or newspapers that haven't been taken in, broken windows or doors ajar that are normally closed. Plus, just their presence on the street can help deter crime.

While I love the beautiful view and the open space around my country home and I do enjoy walking along the country roads despite the lack of sidewalks and the fast-moving traffic, I often tell my husband that eventually, especially when we retire, I'd like to live in a more walkable community so that I can rely on foot power more than gasoline to get around. I'd want walking to be very natural part of my daily routine.

I believe this should be a key consideration for folks who are considering moving after the kids go to college or after they retire. In fact, a recent article in *Modern Maturity* magazine noted that many of their surveyed readers were returning to city life now that their kids were grown. They could give up lawn care and gain access to so many more cultural opportunities, great restaurants, theaters, and so on. And they could walk to their destinations, getting a healthy dose of activity to boot.

# The Program

For this walking program, I want you to become your own Personal Transportation Engineer. I am assuming that you're in good enough shape to walk a couple of miles at a time without becoming overly tired, but that you've been walking those miles on your treadmill, at a health club, or around the neighborhood with no particular destination in mind. Now you're going to start thinking of your walking ability as a transportation asset in addition to being a health necessity. You're going to start to figure out practical and fun ways to work walking into your daily routine. If you're like me, you'll find that walking "to get somewhere" is a very rewarding way to walk, and that distance and time seem like much less effort when you're walking with a particular errand or destination in mind. This is the most natural way to walk—and one that many Americans have forgotten!

First of all, just sit down with a pencil and paper and think about your lifestyle and all the car trips you take during a month. Make a list of your destinations. Most of the trips people take by car are not work-related. They're for shopping, doctor's visits, social visits, religious services, and so on.

Once you have your list, write down next to each destination how much time it takes you to drive there and how many miles you *think* it is. Then get out your map and highlight the routes you would take to walk to any of the destinations that are three miles or less. You may be surprised to see that you greatly overestimated the distance on some trips. We so rarely walk for transportation that I think most people aren't very good at eyeballing distances. I remember on my first walking vacation in England, we'd leave a small village in the morning, and in the afternoon we'd stop on a hilltop for lunch and look back to where we'd just walked from. I was always astounded to see how far we'd come, thinking it looked so much farther away that it actually was!

Your walking route may be quite different from your driving route, since you likely stick to more major roads with your car, but you can zigzag through a neighborhood on foot. Or maybe you have access to a walking path that is even shorter than the route you'd take by car. Also keep in mind that parking your car may make many of your shorter trips a time-consuming headache, and that walking might take even less time and save money.

Be sure to consider the trips you take from your workplace during lunch or breaks, and errands you run on the way home from work. Can you park somewhere on your way home to walk an errand, creating an island of time for you to de-stress before greeting your partner or other family members?

Measure your routes and, using the scale of the map, figure out the approximate distance of each route and multiply that by your walking speed. For instance, if a trip is 1.5 miles and you walk 1 mile in 17 minutes, then it will take you 1.5 × 17 or about 26 minutes to walk there, plus 26 minutes to walk back to your starting point. Write your round-trip times next to each destination in your list.

It might look something like this:

1. Grocery store: 50 minutes round trip

2. Dentist: 40 minutes round trip

3. Veterinarian: 30 minutes round trip (and the dog gets to walk too!)

4. Post office: 20 minutes round trip

5. Ice cream parlor: 30 minutes round trip

6. Work: 60 minutes round trip

7. Train station: 30 minutes round trip

8. Beauty salon: 30 minutes round trip

9. Place of worship: 37 minutes round trip

I'm not saying it's practical for you to act as if you don't own a car and that you have the time to switch all your local car travel to walking trips. But I'm challenging you to take this information and apply it for the next month in the best way that you can, for fun, and see how it works for you.

Get out your calendar or appointment book and look at your schedule for the next thirty days. Using the chart below, pencil in as many walking trips as you feel are workable. See if you can schedule longer walks for the weekend or any time you have more flexibility. If you'd like to walk to the movie theater or to dinner, get your partner involved. You may have to adjust your clothing somewhat, but most people can walk a couple of miles at a comfortable pace without working up a big sweat. And you can wear comfortable shoes or sandals instead of sneakers.

If you're going shopping, see if you can carry your purchases in a backpack. (As a bonus, you'll burn some extra calories.) Or if you're grocery shopping for only one or two people, can you fit your purchases into a personal shopping cart that you can push home easily?

I realize that what I'm suggesting here can require some real advance planning and rearranging of your life. But doesn't it often seem that we're always hurrying here and there in our cars and then wondering when we'll fit in the time to exercise? And wouldn't it be nice to slow down the pace of our lives, so that health-giving, tension-reducing walks become a natural part of it?

On the days when you can't schedule a practical trip walk, you should still pencil in your thirty-minute-minimum-for-health walk on the treadmill or around the neighborhood. Just looking at the juxtaposition of those facts on paper might bring about some revelations about how you spend your time.

Try this for a month and see if it doesn't energize your exercise, bring you into closer contact with your neighbors, allow you to appreciate your town or city in new ways, and spark interest in other walks you might like to take!

| | Monday | Tuesday | Wednesday | Thursday | Friday | Saturday | Sunday |
|---|---|---|---|---|---|---|---|
| **Week 1** | | | | | | | |
| Exercise walk: (minutes) | | | | | | | |
| Errand walk: (minutes) | | | | | | | |
| **Week 2** | | | | | | | |
| Exercise walk: (minutes) | | | | | | | |
| Errand walk: (minutes) | | | | | | | |
| **Week 3** | | | | | | | |
| Exercise walk: (minutes) | | | | | | | |
| Errand walk: (minutes) | | | | | | | |
| **Week 4** | | | | | | | |
| Exercise walk: (minutes) | | | | | | | |
| Errand walk: (minutes) | | | | | | | |
| **Week 5** | | | | | | | |
| Exercise walk: (minutes) | | | | | | | |
| Errand walk: (minutes) | | | | | | | |

# Stress Reduction: Soar Like an Eagle

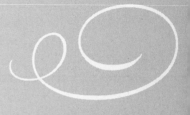

**Use this program if you**
- want to increase the stress-reducing power of your walk;
- are interested in the benefits of meditation but have never been able to sit still long enough to experience them;
- tend to overwork your brain while walking because you use the time to think about problems;
- want to feel more refreshed, alive, and focused during and after your walk.

**What You'll Need:** A watch or stopwatch to time intervals, and a safe, pleasant trail or track where you can walk without having to watch or stop for traffic. Having a tape recorder or friend to read exercises to you can be very helpful when learning the Awakener exercises.

*"Our minds and our bodies hold energy in the form of tension and attention. Release tension and direct attention, and we summon up vast new energy resources."*

—*Gurucharan Singh Khalsa, Ph.D., coauthor of* Breathwalk

*B*reathwalk is a self-help technique, a way to combine the physical activity of walking with specialized breathing patterns and mental focus to bring about, literally, a change in consciousness. It's a moving meditation technique that can help you reduce anxiety and tension. Freed from anxiety and tension, you experience renewed energy and vitality, brighter thoughts, and creative solutions. In their book, *Breathwalk: Breathing Your Way to a Revitalized Body, Mind, and Spirit* (Broadway Books, 2001, New York, NY), Gurucharan Singh Khalsa, Ph.D., and Yogi Bhajan, Ph.D., elaborate on sixteen different styles of Breathwalk, each with a targeted mental, emotional, or spiritual outcome such as reducing depression, accelerating intuition, and improving a sense of relatedness to your partner.

Breathwalk was designed to help people gain control over their mental and emotional states while invigorating and relaxing their bodies with exercise. As Gurucharan explained to me as he introduced me to his work, "Breathwalk gives you the ability to choose your mood."

It makes perfect sense that affecting your breath can affect your mood and mental state. After all, think about how your breath is affected when you feel fear, joy, happiness, or anxiety. Your breathing may become shallow and fast-paced or deeper and slower depending on your emotions. Or it can come in short, explosive bursts when you laugh. That circuitry can work both ways! If you deepen your breathing, you'll feel more relaxed. You don't need to be at the mercy of your emotional reactions. You can take control of your breathing and experience profound benefits. The power of the breath to calm and center has resulted in meditation classes springing up around the country, not just in yoga centers and ashrams, but in hospitals and wellness centers.

Herbert Benson, M.D., founding president of the Mind/Body Medical Institute and associate professor of medicine at Harvard University, distilled essential aspects of meditation into the Relaxation Response technique, a westernized version of eastern techniques. In his forward to *Breathwalk,* Dr. Benson notes that "the benefits for positive mood elevation and enhanced healing are triggered by this combination (of focused attention and rhythmical exercise) and not just by exercise or walking alone."

In my discussions with Gurucharan, we talked about other moving meditation techniques, such as that of the Buddhist monk Thich Nat Hahn, who used a very slow walk with repeated affirmations. Gurucharan remarked that in his work with depressed patients, this slow movement had a similar impact as sitting meditations—many depressed patients felt *more* depressed. Brisk walking is known to lift people's spirits and combat mild to moderate depression. This was part of what lead him and Yogi Bhajan to develop breathing techniques to match a more invigorating walking style.

Adding mindful attention to physical activity is not just holding back random negativity, though that in itself is helpful. A mindful approach to any activity, says Gurucharan, creates openness to new information and an implicit awareness of more than one perspective. During Breathwalk, your mind "is primed for learning, creativity, and getting out of old ruts of thinking and feeling."

After our introductory meeting, I began practicing Breathwalk during my regular morning walks. This was during a pretty stressful period in my work and personal life. My sons were leaving for college, my mother (who lived seventy miles away) needed more help and attention, my work was more demanding, and my husband sometimes felt ignored or left out; in short, I felt pulled in many different directions. Sound familiar?

I found the Breathwalk practice immediately calming. Breathwalk helped me to focus my attention on breathing techniques and mental sounds, rather than drifting from one problem to the next or jumping the gun on my work day, which often resulted in one of two things: I'd stop my walk early, feeling agitated about work I had to get done, or my mind would be so preoccupied and revved up that even if I kept walking for thirty to sixty minutes, my walk would lose much of its power to relax me. I'd feel drained rather than recharged. After a Breathwalk, I'd often find new ideas bubbling to the surface. Now, this often happens for me on any solitary walk, as I'm sure it does for you. But when under stress, I found Breathwalk helped me to stop anxious, negative thoughts which would normally pound at me with every step.

Based on the ancient practice of Kundalini yoga, each Breathwalk has specific physical exercises to support the intentions of the walker. They act like a jump start for your personal battery, to get you headed in the right direction.

A complete Breathwalk has five parts:

*The Awakener:* a series of exercises to give you a quick tune-up

*Alignment:* walking while paying attention to your form and current feelings

*The Breathwalk:* walking while using a specific breathing technique

*Balance:* reconnecting to your surroundings

*Integration:* an "innerwalk" that occurs while you walk slowly or sit quietly and helps you to gain new perspectives from your Breathwalk experience and carry them into your day

Taking all five steps ensures the most complete experience, but you can also use just the breath pattern in a pinch. For instance, if you're getting ready for an important meeting or you're in a hospital waiting to see a friend or family member, just walk up and down the hallway using the breath pattern, and you'll feel yourself getting calmer.

The Breathwalk I'd like to share with you is one of the simplest because the breath matches a natural walking rhythm so well. I suggest practicing the breathing technique a few times while you're sitting with this book, so you can master it now and don't have to try to walk and carry the book around outside!

Sit quietly, feet flat on the floor, hands relaxed in your lap, back straight but not stiff. Take a few relaxed, deep breaths, inhaling and exhaling through your nose. Notice how much air you take in and let flow out.

Now you are going to inhale using four short, segmented breaths, timing them so that on the fourth breath, your lungs are full of air. Then exhale in four short, segmented breaths. It's like taking a short sniff, pausing, then taking another, pausing, another, pausing, and finally one more. It will take a few tries before you figure out how much air you can take in with each breath so you can have four even breaths in and out.

When you inhale, you want the four short breaths to simulate a full breath in, and when you exhale, you want to feel your belly press inward slightly as you expel the last breath, which means you've emptied your lungs pretty well.

Try it a few times. You may find that you feel a little dizzy because you're not used to getting so much oxygen. That's okay. Just stop for a few minutes and then try again. The dizziness will subside.

After you feel comfortable with the breathing pattern, try walking in place as you take the breaths. For each short breath, take one step. So it's step/inhale, step/inhale, step/inhale, step/inhale, in unison, on the in breath, and step/exhale, step/exhale, step/exhale, step/exhale on the out breath. You may find it easier to simply go for a short walk, walking naturally and matching the four/four segmented breath to your pace.

For additional mental focus, you can add what is called the primal sound scale to your walk. As you inhale and exhale, mentally recite "Sa Ta Na Ma." Each syllable corresponds to a step and a segment of breath. Some people like to press the fingers of their hand one at a time, from index finger to pinkie, to their thumbs in rhythm to their breathing and chanting (Gurucharan calls this finger magic).

That is the core of Breathwalk. At first you can practice using the given technique for just a few minutes a day, as part of your daily walk. Then you can gradually increase the duration and alternate with periods of normal breathing, as described in the workout program that follows.

After a week, you can add the other components, which don't really take much extra time at all. The hardest part is reading about them!

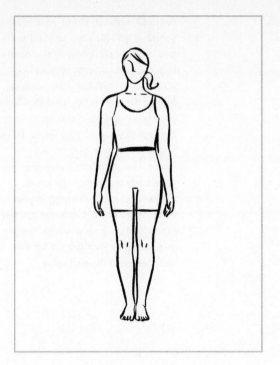

**Awaken:** Standing tall, focus on the end of your nose (gently, don't strain and go cross-eyed!) and center yourself by taking several complete, deep breaths.

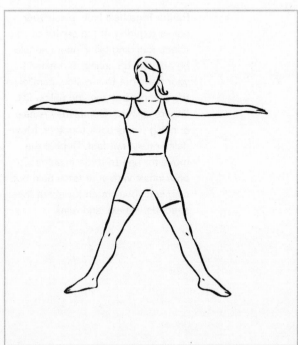

**Star Pose:** Stand with your legs wide apart, arms extended outward, palms facing up. Focus inwardly toward your brow. Begin a long, slow, deep breath, then exhale. Mentally concentrate on feeling your breath in the center of each palm. Sense the connection between your palm and the life around you. Continue for several breaths. To end, inhale deeply and suspend your breath for about five seconds. Then relax your arms and breathe naturally.

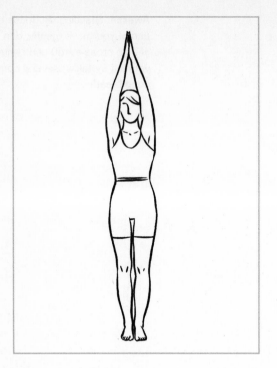

**Arms Overhead:** Bring your legs together and lift your straight arms over your head, bringing the palms together. (Your arms should hug your ears.) Stabilize your posture, feeling strong and grounded. Close your eyes and roll them up to focus through the top of your head. Begin a slow, complete breath. As you inhale, visualize light extending from your body out to the universe. Exhale and relax, drawing in your flash of brilliance. Continue for several breaths. To end, inhale deeply and suspend your breath for five seconds, exhale, and relax.

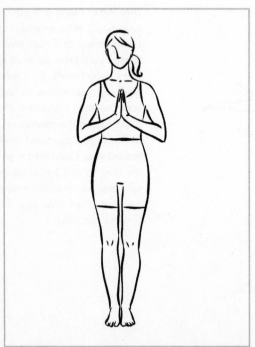

**Palms Together:** Now place your palms together at the center of your chest, standing tall. Fingers should be pointing up. Inhale and extend your arms out to the side, parallel to the ground, but keeping palms flat, fingers upward. Completely exhale, bringing palms back together. Move deliberately, not fast. Repeat the move for one to three minutes. To end, inhale with your arms held out, suspend your breath for about five seconds, exhale, and relax.

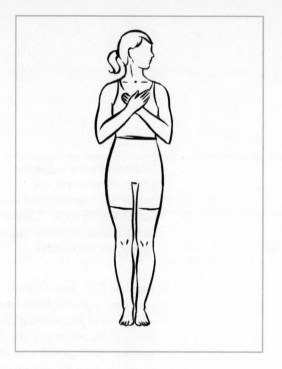

**Crossed Arms:** Standing tall, relax your shoulders and lift your chest slightly. Cross your hands over your chest, right hand over left. Begin deep breathing. As you inhale, turn your head to the left. As you exhale, turn your head to the right. Keep your shoulders relaxed and move deliberately and smoothly. Do not strain. Continue for several breaths. To end, bring your head back to center and inhale, suspend your breath for five seconds, exhale completely, suspend your breath for five seconds, and relax. Notice how you feel.

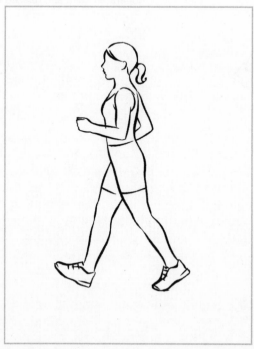

**Align:** Begin walking after these exercises and take some time just to establish a comfortable, relaxed rhythm. Notice how you feel and check yourself for proper posture. Are your shoulders relaxed? Head over shoulders? Pelvis supporting your upper body? (Remember, press your belly button toward your spine to bring your pelvis into alignment.)

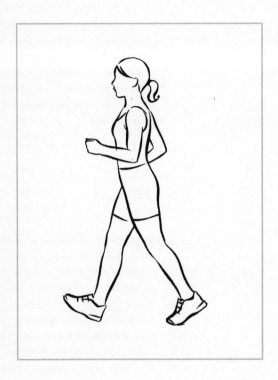

**Vitalize:** Use the suggested breathing pattern of four segmented breaths in and four out, called the Eagle. Add the primal sounds and finger tapping as you feel comfortable.

**Balance:** Cool down by slowing your pace gradually. Notice the world around you, allowing your sense to expand as you focus on your surroundings with your newly generated calm and relaxed energy.

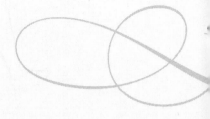

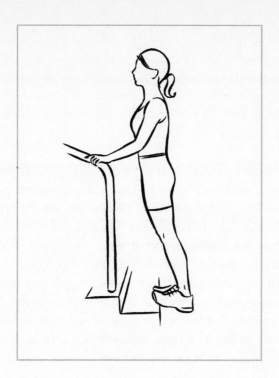

**Stretch:** Take a moment to stretch your calves, hamstrings, and shins.

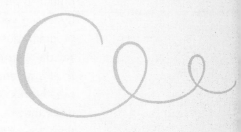

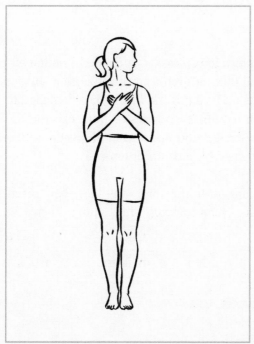

**Integrate with an Innerwalk:** Sit or stand quietly for two to five minutes. As you breathe in and out, feel the surface of your skin breathe with you. Imagine your breath forming a bubble, a skin of breath all around you that is very sensitive. Let all sounds, feelings, thoughts, smells, and tastes come into your bubble. Imagine this bubble extending out in all directions, as far as you can. Rest quietly in the center of your bubble.

To end, inhale deeply, suspend your breath for five seconds, and release. Inhale, stretch your arms up, and release. Move on to the rest of your day taking this feeling of calm centeredness with you.

## The 4-Week Breathwalk Program

Morning is a great time for a revitalizing Breathwalk—or any walk, for that matter. Sometimes it feels like morning is the only time we can control; it may be the only part of the day that what's important to us doesn't get pushed aside. But the right time for you may be noon, afternoon, or evening. Adapt the program as necessary.

**Note:** I designed this program based on my own experience with the Breathwalk program and my sense of what beginners who have not experienced yoga or breathing techniques will feel comfortable doing. I'll ease you into the program by having you practice unfamiliar techniques and then add to them. While my program closely parallels the original design, it does not include all of the Kundalini stretches and more esoteric aspects of the teaching.

If, at any time, you feel dizzy during the breathing techniques, just relax and breathe normally. People trying this technique tend to hyperventilate at first, while they're experimenting to find the proper depth of inhalation and exhalation. You're also probably getting a lot more oxygen than you're used to, just taking deeper breaths! Think of it as rinsing your brain!

## Week 1

Prepare by scouting your area for a pleasant, fairly level, continuous pathway to walk. A park trail, rail-trail, or even a track in pleasant surroundings is best. It's difficult to focus on breath work when you're looking out for cars or stumbling over rough terrain. Keep notes on your experience, and rate your feeling of anxiety or stress before and after each session, with one being feeling relaxed and ten being very anxious or tense.

*Monday:* Begin by reading over the directions and then practicing the 4/4 breath technique for several minutes while sitting. Then take a brisk 15-minute walk.

**ANXIETY LEVELS BEFORE:** 1 2 3 4 5 6 7 8 9 10 **AFTER:** 1 2 3 4 5 6 7 8 9 10

*Tuesday:* Take a brisk 15-minute walk and play with the 4/4 breath, matching the segments to your step. It may take some experimentation to get the hang of filling your lungs and emptying them fully. Do not try to do the technique continuously. Just play with it for a few minutes. Then relax. Then try again. (Try not to walk in a hilly area. Until you get the hang of the technique, it's best to walk on the flat, where your breathing stays more even.)

ANXIETY LEVELS BEFORE: 1 2 3 4 5 6 7 8 9 10 AFTER: 1 2 3 4 5 6 7 8 9 10

*Wednesday:* Take a brisk 15-minute walk and try the 4/4 pattern for a minute or two, matching the breaths with the mental sounds, Sa, Ta, Na, Ma, as you walk. It's fine to say them under your breath, too, if that helps. Remember the finger magic! Relax and walk normally for a few minutes, then start the pattern again. Repeat.

ANXIETY LEVELS BEFORE: 1 2 3 4 5 6 7 8 9 10 AFTER: 1 2 3 4 5 6 7 8 9 10

*Thursday:* Feeling comfortable with the 4/4 breathing? Try this interval pattern: After warming up for a few minutes, do 3 minutes of 4/4 (Eagle) breathing, then 5 minutes of normal breathing. Repeat 3 times for about a 30-minute walk.

ANXIETY LEVELS BEFORE: 1 2 3 4 5 6 7 8 9 10 AFTER: 1 2 3 4 5 6 7 8 9 10

*Friday:* Repeat Thursday's workout.

ANXIETY LEVELS BEFORE: 1 2 3 4 5 6 7 8 9 10 AFTER: 1 2 3 4 5 6 7 8 9 10

*Saturday:* Find a friend or relative who will read the Awakener exercises to you, step by step, as you move through them. (It's hard to read them and do them at the same time!) Or you can make your own audiotape and listen to it. After you practice the Awakeners, take a normal walk. Notice any difference in how you feel.

ANXIETY LEVELS BEFORE: 1 2 3 4 5 6 7 8 9 10 AFTER: 1 2 3 4 5 6 7 8 9 10

*Sunday:* Rest, walk with a friend, bike, hike, or do some other playful activity.

## Week 2

**Monday:** Practice the Awakener exercises, then begin your walk. Align, Vitalize, Balance, and stretch your calves and hamstrings afterward. Try this pattern: 3 minutes Eagle, 5 minutes normal, 3 minutes Eagle, 5 minutes normal, 5 minutes Eagle, 3 minutes normal.

ANXIETY LEVELS BEFORE: 1 2 3 4 5 6 7 8 9 10   AFTER: 1 2 3 4 5 6 7 8 9 10

**Tuesday:** Repeat Monday's practice.

ANXIETY LEVELS BEFORE: 1 2 3 4 5 6 7 8 9 10   AFTER: 1 2 3 4 5 6 7 8 9 10

**Wednesday:** Repeat Monday's practice, using these intervals: Eagle for 3 minutes, normal breathing for 5 minutes, Eagle for 5, normal for 3, Eagle for 5, normal for 3.

ANXIETY LEVELS BEFORE: 1 2 3 4 5 6 7 8 9 10   AFTER: 1 2 3 4 5 6 7 8 9 10

**Thursday:** Repeat Wednesday's practice.

ANXIETY LEVELS BEFORE: 1 2 3 4 5 6 7 8 9 10   AFTER: 1 2 3 4 5 6 7 8 9 10

**Friday:** Repeat Wednesday's practice.

ANXIETY LEVELS BEFORE: 1 2 3 4 5 6 7 8 9 10   AFTER: 1 2 3 4 5 6 7 8 9 10

**Saturday:** If possible, find a friend with whom you can share the Breathwalk experience. Remember, this can be playful, not overly serious. Share the Awakener exercises and the breath pattern and take a walk together. Share your experiences. Enjoy your surroundings. It's okay to talk together during the normal breathing phase. Strict compliance with timed intervals isn't necessary. Carry a little bell if you like and practice the Eagle breath for a few minutes, then ring the bell to signal regular breathing. Teaching someone else is often the best way to learn to integrate new things into your own life!

ANXIETY LEVELS BEFORE: 1 2 3 4 5 6 7 8 9 10   AFTER: 1 2 3 4 5 6 7 8 9 10

**Sunday:** Rest, walk with a friend, bike, hike, or do some other playful activity.

# Week 3

**Monday:** Make time today to perform the whole Breathwalk ritual: Awakener exercises, Alignment, Vitalize, Balance, Stretch, and Integrate. Note your feelings. Use the following intervals: 3 Eagle, 5 normal, 5 Eagle, 3 normal, 10 Eagle, 1 normal.

ANXIETY LEVELS BEFORE: 1 2 3 4 5 6 7 8 9 10   AFTER: 1 2 3 4 5 6 7 8 9 10

**Tuesday:** Repeat Monday's program.

ANXIETY LEVELS BEFORE: 1 2 3 4 5 6 7 8 9 10   AFTER: 1 2 3 4 5 6 7 8 9 10

**Wednesday:** Repeat Monday's program, but experiment with a different time of day. While a morning Breathwalk is an excellent way to start the day, you may feel more relaxed and renewed if you practice just before dinner or lunch, or in the early evening.

ANXIETY LEVELS BEFORE: 1 2 3 4 5 6 7 8 9 10   AFTER: 1 2 3 4 5 6 7 8 9 10

**Thursday:** Repeat Monday's program. If you find yourself becoming tense or anxious during the day, take a break and do some Eagle breathing for 5 to 10 minutes, even if you have to do it inside your office building or around the block. If you're caring for someone in a wheelchair or stroller, take him or her along for the ride!

ANXIETY LEVELS BEFORE: 1 2 3 4 5 6 7 8 9 10   AFTER: 1 2 3 4 5 6 7 8 9 10

**Friday:** Repeat Monday's program, but try to find a new path or trail to enjoy.

ANXIETY LEVELS BEFORE: 1 2 3 4 5 6 7 8 9 10   AFTER: 1 2 3 4 5 6 7 8 9 10

**Saturday:** Find a buddy again this week and take a Breathwalk together. Notice if this type of mind/body exercise helps you to feel more connected, even without speaking to each other. If you prefer to let the Awakener exercises go, that's fine. Share as much as you feel comfortable with.

ANXIETY LEVELS BEFORE: 1 2 3 4 5 6 7 8 9 10   AFTER: 1 2 3 4 5 6 7 8 9 10

**Sunday:** Rest, play, relax, sing, kayak or canoe, bike, work on a puzzle, try some new yoga poses, or visit with friends and family.

## Week 4

Are you getting comfortable with your Breathwalk practice? Hopefully, you are feeling the positive effects of this mind/body/spirit approach to walking. Continue on with the full program, charting your daily walks and feelings. For more information about Breathwalk or to work with an instructor, go to www.breathwalk.com. There are also teacher trainings available.

**Monday:** Take the time to perform the whole Breathwalk ritual: Awakener exercises, Alignment, Vitalize, Balance, Stretch, and Integrate. Note your feelings. Use the following intervals: 3 Eagle, 5 normal, 5 Eagle, 3 normal, 10 Eagle, 1 normal. Continue this program for the rest of the week.

ANXIETY LEVELS BEFORE: 1 2 3 4 5 6 7 8 9 10   AFTER: 1 2 3 4 5 6 7 8 9 10

**Tuesday**

ANXIETY LEVELS BEFORE: 1 2 3 4 5 6 7 8 9 10   AFTER: 1 2 3 4 5 6 7 8 9 10

**Wednesday**

ANXIETY LEVELS BEFORE: 1 2 3 4 5 6 7 8 9 10   AFTER: 1 2 3 4 5 6 7 8 9 10

**Thursday**

ANXIETY LEVELS BEFORE: 1 2 3 4 5 6 7 8 9 10   AFTER: 1 2 3 4 5 6 7 8 9 10

**Friday**

ANXIETY LEVELS BEFORE: 1 2 3 4 5 6 7 8 9 10   AFTER: 1 2 3 4 5 6 7 8 9 10

**Saturday**

ANXIETY LEVELS BEFORE: 1 2 3 4 5 6 7 8 9 10   AFTER: 1 2 3 4 5 6 7 8 9 10

**Sunday:** Rest. Relax and enjoy family and friends. Play, hike, enjoy nature, bird-watch, bike, do some yoga, or listen to music.

# Power Up Your Stride

**Use this program if you'd like to**
- get a better workout for your calves, legs, and buttocks;
- whittle your waist;
- improve your posture;
- flatten your belly while you walk;
- burn more calories;
- walk in a race or other walking event;
- increase your self-esteem.

**What you'll need:**

A nice, smooth walking surface, such as a track or graveled pathway. Sidewalks are fine as long as they aren't broken up or uneven.

You'll also need a very flexible pair of walking shoes. I like New Balance's 110 Racewalker for women. Walking coach Elaine Ward prefers Asics running shoes. The key is a very flexible shoe with a thinner sole so you can flex your foot easily in the heel-toe motion. Hold the shoe in both hands and bend the toe and heel toward the center. The shoe should flex easily.

In addition, you'll want to have a good pair of walking socks that wick away sweat and keep your feet cool, spandex walking shorts (they won't ride up between your legs!), and a baseball cap or visor so you can keep your head tall when facing the sun.

Ready to learn specific walking techniques that can help you walk faster, look taller and slimmer, and give you more of a total-body workout? These techniques are derived from the sport of racewalking, which developed in England more than 400 years ago. But you don't have to race to incorporate them into your walking workout. That's why lots of walking coaches and teachers have coined new names for the activity, such as healthwalking, pacewalking, and heel-toe walking. Despite the different names, they're all derived from racewalking style.

Learning these techniques can be fun and will give you a great workout; at the same time, your walk will become more graceful. It's not always obvious when people are using walking technique, except for the noticeable arm swing with a bend at the elbow. But walkers who use these techniques seem to move faster with very little effort, and you can't quite figure out why when you're with them. I remember my first exposure to heel-toe walkers in

Central Park. We were all warming up together, walking normally, and then the heel-toe walkers started applying their specialized techniques and they just glided away from me, seemingly effortlessly. It didn't seem like their legs were moving any faster than mine, and they weren't taking big, bouncing strides. It seemed almost magical! I remember staring at them as they continued to outdistance me and asking their coach, David Balboa, "How are they *doing* that?" Heel-toe walkers do not have to look weird or wiggly, like some racewalkers. The best heel-toe walkers just look very smooooooth.

Do I use these special techniques all the time? No. Many times I just enjoy a normal, average walking style. But concentrating on form has improved my posture overall, even when I walk to the mailbox. I can see it in photographs, too. I had a much more stooped posture when I was in my thirties than I do now. My shoulders were rounded, my chest caved in, and I looked depressed and frightened (and I was). I stand taller and stronger now, and my posture reflects my inner strength as well.

In fact, I've read a few studies over the years saying that women who used fitness walking techniques boosted their self-esteem. Basically, that was a result of putting their minds to doing something and accomplishing it, or self-efficacy. Perhaps focusing on form was more helpful than stewing about problems when they walked, too. At any rate, count it as an extra bonus as you go about mastering these techniques.

A word of warning: It takes time for your body to adapt to this new form of walking. If you've been walking regularly at a good clip, you will probably have to slow down to master heel-toe walking. You'll be using your muscles in a whole new way. You'll feel tightness in your butt, your calves, and especially your shins. You'll be working more of your torso and bringing your arms and shoulders into play. You'll need to spend a little more time stretching. Heel-toe walking takes some time, but I'd say it's probably one of the best ways to get fit after forty.

I'll outline the techniques below. If you try them and they don't seem to work for you or you feel uncoordinated, try viewing a video to see fitness walking in action. The technique is very subtle, and it can really help to watch someone else doing it. You can also use one of my walking audiotapes: *Swing Your Way to Weight Loss or Power Up Your Stride*. I provide on-the-spot coaching and encouragement for the technique as well as some strengthening exercises and stretches. (For more information on the audiotapes, go to my Web site at www.walkforallseasons.com.)

Stretching becomes ever more important as you beef up your walking technique. Refer to the stretching and yoga sections on pages 30 and 169 for specific information on calf, shin, hamstring, hip, and other stretches.

**Here we go:**

*Stand tall.* Lift your upper body off your lower body as you press your head toward the sky. Let your pelvis shift, dropping your tailbone toward the ground as you press your pubic bone forward, positioning your lower body for optimum support. Practice this in front of a mirror so that you can see how much it changes your profile. A protruding belly disappears instantly! You look taller and slimmer. Relax your shoulders as you lift your chest enough to stand tall without arching your back. If you feel your back arching, press your sternum (breastbone) down slightly. Standing tall should feel great, not painful—but you may tire of it quickly. It takes time to be able to maintain good posture if you've been slouching all your life!

*Find your stride.* The best, most efficient, and least pounding way to walk faster is to take smaller, quicker steps rather than big, bouncing strides. (Big, long strides will work at first, but you're limited in how many steps you can take in a minute, which is known as your turnover rate. Plus, big bouncing strides are tougher on your back, knees, and ankles.) You want one continuous motion of steps, as though you're gliding along. Find your stride by lifting one leg with a bent knee and then dropping your foot straight down, leading with your heel and straightening your knee. That's a good stride length to shoot for.

*Heel-toe roll.* When you step forward, landing on your heel, keep your toes elevated to about a 45-degree angle. Take a minute to do this now. Stand up, step forward, land on your heel, and straighten your leg. Notice that this engages your entire leg, all the way up to your hip. Now take a few steps forward with your normal gait, which is more flat-footed. Notice the difference. Now go back to landing on your heel, and then roll forward on your foot, from heel to toe. (Imagine you have little rockers on the bottom of your shoe.) This is "heel-toe" walking technique. Practice walking around your house using this motion and notice how it feels.

*Walk the imaginary line.* Imagine there's a line down the middle of your walking path. Try to place your feet close to the line as you land on your heel and move forward. This also helps you to extend from the hip, which lengthens your stride in a new way. Most people don't use their hips when they walk. But it needn't be an obvious wiggle. It's a supple motion, with your hips moving forward and back as you glide through your stride.

***Engage your arms.*** By adding a bent-arm swing to your walk, you gain a total-body workout. This motion works your upper and lower arms to some degree, but it also helps drive your hips forward, which works your torso. Bend your arms to a ninety-degree angle and swing them like a pendulum from your shoulders. (Don't punch forward.) Keep your arms close to your body and your hands lightly cupped, like you're holding a raw egg you don't want to break. Drive your elbows back, till your hand swings alongside your hip, but not behind your back. Then allow your arms to swing forward, bringing your cupped fist no higher than mid-chest (nipple level). Don't swing your arms across the front of your body. Practice your arm swing standing in front of a mirror, so you know what it feels like to practice within the correct range of motion. You will feel your hips start to move as you swing your arms. Go with that motion! Release your hips and let them swivel around your spine, forward and back.

Some people think their arms are driving their workout, but that's not really so. They're accentuating it. Your power is coming from your hips, legs, and feet. Swinging your arms forward and back can help you get more hip rotation and a nice feeling of coordinated rhythm to your walk.

Remember to stay tall, pressing up through the crown of your head. Keep your core strong by keep your pelvis properly positioned, with your tailbone toward the ground and your pubic bone pushed forward slightly. (Suki Munsell, Ph.D., founder of the former Dynamic Walking Institute in California, and one of my teachers, liked to say, "Belly button to backbone!" It's a very effective visualization that helps you keep a strong core and tucked pelvis.) If you've suffered from a sore back or sciatic pain after walking, you may find that soreness disappear as you strengthen your core and put less pressure on your lower back. Yippee!

## Your Workout

After practicing these techniques in front of the mirror, which will seem simple enough, you may go outside and try to master them all at once and feel completely discombobulated! That's natural. It's best to work on them one at a time, gradually trying the new movements and putting them together. I've outlined a 4-week workout schedule to help you. It's designed for people who have already mastered a basic 30-minutes-a-day, most days of the week, walking regimen. I've also added a couple of exercises that will help strengthen your shins and stretch you out as you master the new movement. Remember, don't grit your teeth! Focus, but relax. Picture yourself gliding. Imagine you're floating along. Stay light on your feet. Enjoy!

# Week 1

**Monday:** Warm up for 5 to 10 minutes at a comfortable pace. Stop and stretch your calves and shins. Resume walking and focus only on standing tall, pelvis tucked under, pubic bone pushed slightly forward. Keep your shoulders relaxed. Breathe deeply by expanding your rib cage (rather than breathing deeply into your belly) while keeping your abdominal muscles engaged. When you get tired, relax and walk normally for a few minutes, then return to your "tall" posture. Walk this way for about 15 minutes. Cool down (walk at a slower pace) for 5 to 10 minutes. Stretch.

**Notes:** How long were you able to maintain your posture?

_____

_____

_____

How did you feel?

_____

_____

**Tuesday:** Warm up for 5 to 10 minutes, focusing on standing tall. To strengthen you shins and calves for heel-toe walking, try this: Walk on your heels, with your toes pointing up, for about 20 paces. Then walk normally. Then walk on your toes for another 20 paces. Repeat. Now apply the heel-toe technique, moving slowly enough to focus on the whole motion—landing your heel, rolling through the midline of your foot to your toe. You're retraining your muscles, so don't try to go fast. You'll probably feel your shins get tired fairly quickly. When you do, walk normally and pick up your pace to your normal gait.

Go back and forth between heel-toe walking and normal walking for 20 minutes. Cool down and stretch your calves, shins, and hamstrings.

*Notes:* How many steps did you take before your shins felt tired or started to burn?

_____

_____

*Wednesday:* Repeat Tuesday's workout. As you get more comfortable with the heel-toe technique, remember to concentrate on standing tall, too.

*Thursday:* Warm up for 5 to 10 minutes. Try some heel walking and tippy-toe walking again. Then focus on your posture, standing tall. Begin the heel-toe technique. Today, focus on your hips a little more. Let them move forward with each step, in a swivel-type motion. As you do, you'll notice your arms automatically begin to swing more, too. Just let them swing naturally. Go back and forth between heel-toe and normal walking in a way that feels comfortable to you. Don't force it—you'll just get really sore shins! Right now, you're simply getting accustomed to the technique. Continue for about 20 minutes, cool down for 5, and stretch.

*Friday:* Add your arms to the workout. Bend your elbows to about 90 degrees and let them swing naturally from your shoulders. Some people think too hard when doing this and starting swinging their arms out of sync, moving their right arm forward when their right leg steps forward. If you find yourself doing this, stop. Start walking heel-to-toe and let your arms swing naturally. The left arm comes forward when the right leg comes forward. After you've established your rhythm, then bend your arms. Since you're not going too fast yet, there's no need to pump your arms fast. Just keep in rhythm with your legs. Your arms may get tired. Alternate between the technique and normal walking in a way that feels comfortable to you. Cool down for 5 minutes and stretch.

*Saturday:* Put it all together. You've given yourself a chance to play with each part of the technique. Repeat Friday's workout, alternating between heel-toe and normal walking technique. Focus on staying tall and allowing your hips to swivel naturally forward and back. To establish a comfortable rhythm and stay light and flexible, it can be helpful to imagine yourself dancing. If you concentrate too hard, you'll get rigid and inflexible. Listening to upbeat music can help, too. Remember, you're not marching—you're gliding. Your hips and waist may feel sore or tight from this new effort. In addition to stretching your calves, shins, and hamstrings, add hip stretches and side stretches.

*Sunday:* Take a day off. Feel free to do some other activity that gets you off your feet, like biking or swimming or kayaking. Or just relax.

## Week 2

Do your shin strengtheners. Warm up. Apply heel-toe technique at intervals that are comfortable for you. Begin to speed up a little bit with the new technique and see how that feels. If your shins burn too much, back off. If your shins are feeling sore, stop and stretch your shins and calves during the workout. You can also ice them after the workout. You may want to alternate days of heel-toe walking with regular walking. Always stretch afterward.

*Monday:* _____

_____

_____

*Tuesday:* _____

_____

_____

*Wednesday:* _____

_____

*Thursday:* _____

_____

_____

*Friday:* _____

_____

_____

*Saturday:* _____

_____

_____

*Sunday:* _____

_____

## Week 3

There's no telling how long it's going to take you to adapt to this new form. Your shins may be very slow in warming up to this new technique, and it may take weeks or even months before you can walk for a full 30 minutes using it. You're still getting great benefits by using more muscles. Relax and enjoy the glide. When you're doing it right, you'll notice that there's no bounce in your step. Your head is staying level, not bobbing up and down. You're getting less impact in your feet and knees than you do with regular walking. As you begin to add some speed during your heel-toe intervals, focus on driving your elbows back during your arm swings. This will automatically help your hip extend forward, and your stride will lengthen. You'll notice your speed increasing because of the longer stride, even though your feet are not moving faster.

*Monday:* _____

_____

_____

*Tuesday:* _____

_____

_____

*Wednesday:* _____

_____

_____

**Thursday:** _____

_____

_____

**Friday:** _____

_____

_____

**Saturday:** _____

_____

_____

**Sunday:** _____

_____

## Week 4

Focusing on the push-off from your back leg adds more power to your walk. However, it also creates a completely different feeling of effort from what you have been doing so far. Except when training for a 5K and feeling ambitious, I rarely use much push-off technique. I'm happy just to focus on increasing my number of steps per minute (turnover rate) and my arm swing to work out my whole body, glide along, and burn more calories. But if you'd like an even more strenuous workout and more muscle toning and speed, focus on pushing off from your back foot. This is where heel-toe walking or race-walking starts to get closer to running, because pushing off will propel you upward as well as forward to some degree. It will increase your stride length because in order to push, you'll have to leave your back foot on the ground a little bit longer; you'll come up on the toes of your back foot, and your front foot will land farther out. Give it a try. It's a very powerful walk. You'll need to be more vigilant about stretching. Be careful not to overdue it; you could strain muscles or create a pounding effect if you're not careful. Try to keep your stride smooth and glide-like.

*Monday:* _____

_____

_____

*Tuesday:* _____

_____

_____

*Wednesday:* _____

_____

_____

*Thursday:* _____

_____

_____

*Friday:* _____

_____

_____

*Saturday:* _____

_____

_____

*Sunday:* _____

_____

If you're interested in pursuing heel-toe or racewalk technique further, there are lots of books and videos out there to help you. They include many more stretches, strengtheners, and exercises to help you improve form and flexibility. Help from a coach is probably invaluable. Some walking coaches offer video coaching: You send them a video of your walk, and they critique your form for you. As with any endeavor, you can spend lots of time improving your technique, leading to greater speed, strength, and endurance.

# Power Up Plus: Walking with Tools

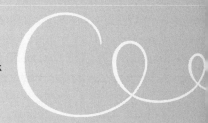

**Use this program if you want to**

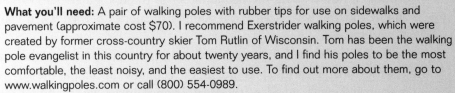

- burn more calories without necessarily increasing your pace
- get a total-body workout
- firm up and tone your upper arms and abdominal muscles while you walk
- try something new to avoid boredom
- alleviate tension in your upper back and shoulders
- ease arthritic knees or feet.

**What you'll need:** A pair of walking poles with rubber tips for use on sidewalks and pavement (approximate cost $70). I recommend Exerstrider walking poles, which were created by former cross-country skier Tom Rutlin of Wisconsin. Tom has been the walking pole evangelist in this country for about twenty years, and I find his poles to be the most comfortable, the least noisy, and the easiest to use. To find out more about them, go to www.walkingpoles.com or call (800) 554-0989.

You'll also need a PowerBelt from the Walker's Warehouse. It comes with a video and two powerpaks for increased resistance. The belt fits up to a 48-inch waist and costs around $80. To order, go to www.walkerswarehouse.com or call (888) 972-9255. (It's not easy to find these products in stores. They're available almost exclusively through mail order.)

Finally, you'll need a continuous walking trail in a park or on a track or along country roads where you feel safe. Walking city sidewalks with curbs and dealing with stop-and-go traffic isn't going to help you get a great workout.

*W*hen I first started to write about walking for *Prevention* magazine, I was pretty much of a purist. I thought walking outside, taking in the beauty of nature, was the optimum way to exercise, and that gadgets detracted from that experience. I knew that hand weights could cause tendinitis in the shoulders or wrists and throw off your normal gait, so I advised against using them.

So when I was first introduced to tools like the PowerBelt and Exerstriders (walking poles), I was pretty disdainful. Why mess with a good thing? Besides, I thought they looked kind of silly. That was when I was in my thirties and could eat pretty much what I wanted and stay thin.

But in my forties, as I started to gain weight, I could see I was going to have to do more to battle the bulge. Over the years, I'd seen many people put out heroic efforts to lose weight, taking all kinds of classes, walking, weight lifting, and so on, only to gain it back when, for whatever reasons, they could no longer walk or run that far, make it to the gym to lift weights, bike that many miles, or make it to that extra aerobics class. So suddenly, these power tools began to make a lot more sense. *They don't require more time.* They make your current workout more powerful.

I try to use these tools whenever they make sense for my workout. They no longer seem silly! They can boost the calorie burn of a walk *between 20 and 50 percent*, depending on your fitness level and how vigorously and continuously you use them. Yet they don't feel as strenuous as pushing your walking speed past the fifteen-minute mile mark because the activity is spread out over more muscle groups. The effect can be like turning your walk into a run, without the pounding. Plus, you're toning your arms and building muscle, which can mean additional calories burned when you're not working out.

The PowerBelt and Exerstrider walking poles are similar in that they bring the upper body into play. But they're certainly different in the way you use them and which muscles they target. I notice tightening around my torso (oblique muscles) with both tools, but walking with poles gives my back and abdominal muscles a better workout. With a PowerBelt, I can also use race-walk technique and speed up my walk, too. I know walkers who love one or the other. I like to use both. Certain walks just seem perfect for the PowerBelt, especially on flat surfaces, so I like using it on the walking track across the street from my house. When I'm going to walk around the very hilly neighborhood where I live, I prefer to use the poles. It's really easy to push the poles into the ground going uphill and get an even better workout while taking some of the stress off my lower body. Coming downhill, they can take some of the stress off your knees. Poles also provide me with a sense of security from stray dogs. (You can offer the pole, instead of your arm, if they attack you.)

One study showed that when done regularly, walking with poles eased neck pain and shoulder tension in office workers, probably by providing greater blood circulation to those areas (though just getting out and exercising may help also). And over the course of a mile, walking with poles has been shown to reduce the accumulated force on the lower body by *about six tons.*

A few years ago, my older sister went to Finland to experience a new walking pole on the market and undergo some fitness testing. The company hooked her up to all kinds of monitoring equipment and had her walk on a treadmill with and without poles, at the same speed. The monitoring devices showed that while she was walking with poles, she was using more energy, her heart was beating faster, and she was burning more calories, but she reported that walking with poles didn't seem any harder. I thought that was pretty cool. Burn more calories, without feeling more physically stressed. Walking fast can be perceived as fun, but many people say it feels too hard. Using these tools can provide a way to pump up your workout without pooping *you* out.

That said, there's still the "foolish factor." The use of these tools is still not widespread in the United States. If you're going to use them, you're probably going to stand out. If you're not the kind of person who likes to draw attention to yourself, these tools may not be for you. But I've found that many women gain steadily in confidence as they age, and like me, you may not give a hoot what other people think about your new power tools. If someone asks you, "What happened to the snow?" when you're out with your walking poles, just smile. If a passerby points at you while you're pumping your Powerbelt, stand taller and pump a little harder! You go, Girl!

## Walking with Poles

Most walking poles come with a full set of instructions and a video that shows you how to use them to best advantage, so there's no point in my trying to duplicate that information here. I prefer the Exerstrider brand to others because of their simplicity, sturdiness, and lack of vibration when walking. Some newer poles come with an attached glove or hand-grip apparatus that allows you to release the pole on the backward swing, as you would when cross-country skiing. But I just find them confusing (which hand in which glove, where do my fingers go, and so on). Plus, there is really no reason to release the pole from a relaxed grip.

Telescoping versions are helpful if you like to travel with your poles or if you share them with someone else, as they need to be adjusted for your height. And there is a version that is more adaptable to a variety of terrains you might encounter when hiking.

In general, you can use your walking poles on asphalt, sidewalk, track, or smooth trail. Hiking poles are another matter; they're really designed to assist you in climbing and descending hills or walking around rough terrain. Walking with poles, as opposed to hiking, is a distinct, total-body exercise activity you can do every day. It doesn't take long to master the technique. You'll be off and striding in no time. (See image on following page.)

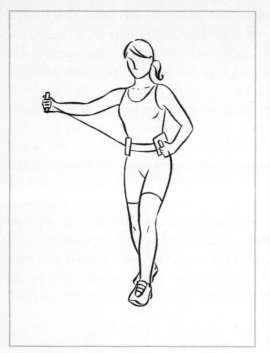
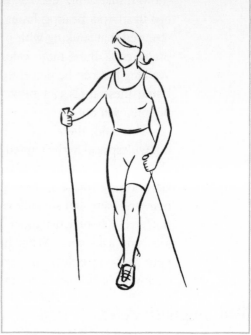

## Walking with the PowerBelt

The PowerBelt is an exercise device you strap around your waist. It has handles attached to cords that coil around a housing on the belt, allowing you to pump your arms back and forth as the cords wind and unwind, providing resistance to your arm swing. Unlike hand weights, you don't have to grip the handles hard (which can actually raise blood pressure). And if your arms get tired, you just let go of the handles and they snap into place at your waist. Your range of motion is similar to the arm pumping you do when racewalking; in fact, the Powerbelt helps keep your arms in the proper alignment. (It's hard to cross over your chest when you're using the PowerBelt. Plus, the cords help to draw your elbows straight back, and you can't push the handles behind your back.)

While just pumping your arms increases calorie burn and helps to tone your upper arms and torso, the Powerbelt adds resistance to make that effect more, well, powerful! And it gives you something to play with. Some of you may feel less self-conscious pumping your arms with a Powerbelt than without one.

Another advantage of the Powerbelt is that it's easy to use on the tread-mill when it's too cold or too hot to walk outside. The video that accompanies it shows you a treadmill workout where you can use the resistance cords in a variety of moves to get even more of a workout for your upper body.

## Why Both?

Can you get by with just one power tool? Of course. But I really like using both. You might find one serves you much better than the other. If you have painful knees or balance problems, for instance, or you're really interested in increasing core strength without doing crunches, then the poles are definitely your first choice. Otherwise, you won't know which one you prefer until you try them. If someone you know uses one, ask if you can borrow it for a walk. Most walkers I know love sharing their enthusiasm for their power tools with their friends.

Finally, before I present my power tools workout program, I'd like to add a word about stretching. Power tools add extra stress to your upper body, so be sure to add the following yoga stretches after your workout: Eagle, Cow Pose with strap, and Knee Down Twist. (See the Special Bonus Yoga Section, beginning on page 169.)

## The 4-Week Power Up Plus Workout

This workout schedule is set for one power tool. If you have both, repeat each week with the alternate tool, creating an 8-week program, so you give your body a chance to adapt to each technique without rushing it. Be ready to kiss your flabby arms good-bye!

Remember to warm up and cool down for at least 5 minutes before and after your workout. When using the poles, don't press down hard, and use a very relaxed grip. With the Powerbelt, just release the handles for warm-ups and cooldowns.

## Week 1

**Monday/Wednesday/Friday:** Walk with poles or the PowerBelt for 20 minutes. Stay at a comfortable pace. You'll notice that your heart starts pumping harder, even though you're not walking faster. Stay within a comfortable intensity, where you can easily carry on a conversation.

**Poles:** Remember to maintain good posture. Don't lean forward from your waist. Use a relaxed grip and don't focus on putting too much pressure on the downward thrust of the poles. Focus on getting into a rhythm and getting comfortable with your new equipment.

*PowerBelt:* Start with the least amount of resistance (no added powerpaks). Swing your arms until they feel tired. Then release the handles till any discomfort fades. When you feel ready, grab them again. Alternate back and forth throughout the workout.

*Tuesday/Thursday/Saturday:* Walk without power tools for 30 minutes or more (assuming you started this program from a baseline of almost daily 30-minute walks).

*Sunday:* Rest.

---
---
---
---
---

## Week 2

*Monday/Wednesday/Friday:* Walk for 20 minutes with your poles or your Powerbelt.

*Poles:* This week, focus on planting the poles very lightly and then pressing down and back with a little more effort. Be careful not to slam the pole into the ground, which can lead to injury. Improper technique could cause inflammation in your wrists, elbows, or shoulders. Pushing on the poles with as much force as is comfortable for you, after they have landed softly, will yield the maximum results.

*PowerBelt:* Keep alternating between using the handles and allowing them to retract so that you can return to just normal arm swinging when your arms tire. Pushing through a little bit of "burn" is fine, but don't overdo it. If at any time burn turns to pain, drop the handles and finish your workout without them.

*Tuesday/Thursday/Saturday:* Revert to your regular 30-minute walk.

*Sunday:* Rest.

_____

_____

_____

_____

# Week 3

*Monday/Wednesday/Friday:* Walk for 30 minutes with your poles or your PowerBelt.

*Poles:* You should be feeling pretty comfortable with the rhythm by now and pushing down firmly on the poles, activating large core strength and back muscles. Be sure to keep a natural, comfortable stride length. Using the poles can tend to lengthen your stride, but keeping a comfortable stride length actually results in more upper-body muscle-conditioning resistance.

*PowerBelt:* Continue in the same pattern of alternating the Powerbelt with your regular arm swing, steadily decreasing the length of your breaks. When you can walk for 30 minutes without taking a break, you may want to step up to the next resistance level, at which time you should begin alternating again. Or focus on heel-toe walking technique to add power to your lower-body workout.

*Tuesday/Thursday/Saturday:* Revert to your regular 30-minute walk.

*Sunday:* Rest.

_____

_____

_____

_____

# Week 4

**Monday/Wednesday/Friday:** Walk for 30 minutes with your poles or your Powerbelt.

**Poles:** Change your route, if you can, to include some rolling hills. You'll love the way it feels to move uphill with them!

**PowerBelt:** If you're using the handles continuously, try throwing in some of the other moves once in a while. Lift the handles out to the sides and over your head while you walk. Try it with your palms facing up and facing down. Also, try extending the handles straight out in front of you at the same time, squeezing your shoulders as you press forward. Have fun with them!

**Tuesday/Thursday/Saturday:** Revert to your regular workout or try using your power tool on any or all of these days. It's up to you. Just listen to the signals from your body. If you start to hurt anywhere, back off. Once you adapt to these tools, though, you may want to use them all the time. Experiment with speed. Can you pick up your pace a little? (But be careful with the poles. If you start walking too fast, you may not be able to push off on the poles as firmly, thereby compromising your upper-body workout. Rutlin himself walks a 16- to 17-minute mile and gets great results!) Stay within your target rate by monitoring your breathing; if you can sing, you're not pushing hard enough. If you can't carry on a conversation because you're gasping for breath, cut back.

**Sunday:** Rest.

---
---
---
---

**PROGRAM 6**

# Ramp Up for a 5K Race

**Use this program if you'd like to**

• super-tone your legs, hips, and buns and trim your waist;

• burn more calories and fat;

• energize your program with a goal;

• power up your fitness and gain oodles of energy;

• boost your confidence and self-esteem;

• find your inner speed demon and impress friends and family;

• enjoy race camaraderie and discover your competitive fire!

**What You'll Need:** A good pair of flexible walking shoes, especially if you're going to use heel-toe walking technique. (See page 67.) A heavy, stiff walking shoe will tire you more quickly and be hard on your shins. Also invest in some great pairs of socks, and find yourself some inspiring workout clothes—shirts and shorts that wick away sweat and dry quickly.

Buy a stopwatch to time your intervals. (Check your local sporting goods or running store.) I have one that I wear around my neck, made by Everlast ($20). It's easy to read and the buttons are big. It even has a little pen attached and note pad inside. You may prefer something you wear on your wrist. But I find lots of wristwatches too complicated and hard to read, especially if I'm wearing my contacts instead of my trifocals.

*I*f you were born before the 1960s, there's a good chance you never participated in serious athletic events in junior high, high school, or even college. Unlike your daughters or nieces who've had full access to team sports and serious athletic pursuits throughout their lives, you may have missed out on that wonderful opportunity to test your strength and endurance and feel the true grit of your competitive instincts. In my own high school, the most athletic pursuit for girls supported by school funding was cheerleading. Girls with athletic talent and drive were left to their own devices to achieve athletic goals and spent early morning hours or weekends training with coaches paid by their parents.

Those of us who considered ourselves tomboys played intramural sports, meaning we played each other, but not other schools. But the focus of these sessions was play, with little emphasis on practice or skill building or an ethic of constant improvement, so few of us took those games seriously. I remember being kicked off an intramural basketball team by a junior high school gym teacher for "giggling too much."

Have you ever marveled at those who've had the discipline to train their bodies for the sake of a sport (including your own sons or daughters)? Many mature women have no idea what it's like to push themselves hard athletically, to test their physical limits beyond what's necessary for day-to-day living or better health. From that side of the playing field, the effort to get fit or super-fit may seem like pure torture. Why bother?

The rewards are there, and they don't necessarily have anything to do with winning. Dramatically increasing your fitness can feel like *nothing you have ever experienced before.* The feeling of living large, in the moment, with every limb enlivened, your senses heightened, and your confidence surging, can give you a whole new perspective on what you are capable of physically, emotionally, and mentally. You may begin to understand, appreciate, admire—even identify with—athletes of any sport for the first time. You can gain a new and deeper perspective of their world, and it can leave you expanded and invigorated in ways you cannot understand until you've tasted athletic effort from your own sweat-drenched brow. Trying to communicate what experiencing more-than-average fitness is like to a person who's never sought physical prowess is kind of like trying to explain what orgasm feels like to the uninitiated. You really won't know until you get there.

Training for a 5K (3.1 miles) walk can be fun, motivating, and challenging, and it can produce all the benefits stated above. Of course, you can moderate how much or how little you put toward the effort. But the more you get into the athletic spirit, the more you'll gain. And that doesn't mean you have to commit to this high level of performance for the rest of your walking life. It may be just a high-level interlude, something to inspire and motivate you for a few months or a few years. That's fine. Your life, your needs, your health and fitness goals will shift according to myriad circumstances. But if you're in good health, without any injuries or serious health challenges, now may be the time to ramp it up for fun and fitness. Here's a step-by-step guide to help you plan, train for, and walk your first 5K event. It just may turn you on to a whole new world of walking.

## Are You Ready for This?

To begin this training program, you should already be meeting the basic requirements of walking for health, which means walking at a moderately brisk pace (at least a twenty-minute-per-mile pace) for thirty minutes most days of the week. With that kind of fitness level, walking for an hour should be no problem, so mark off a 3.1-mile course somewhere, using the odometer on your car, or using accurate park maps, and walk it at a moderately brisk pace, a pace where you feel comfortable. If you're walking at a 20-minute-per-mile pace, it will take you a little over an hour.

*Note: You should be walking briskly most days of the week for thirty minutes, for about two months, before you can begin this training program.* If you try to hop into this training program without mastering the basics, you run the risk of injury, discouragement, or burnout. Athletic walking at faster speeds is simple enough, but it's not easy. Shaving seconds off a twenty- or fifteen-minute mile is challenging, and walking faster than a twelve-minute mile (which can burn as much as 500 calories in an hour) can feel more strenuous than jogging, because at that speed, walking becomes biomechanically inefficient. You may feel like your feet are just begging to lift off the ground, and you have to use special techniques to go faster while keeping one foot on the ground at all times. While jogging and running are certainly legitimate pursuits, there is far greater risk of injury to your feet, ankles, knees, back, and hips, especially as you age.

Whittling your time down to faster speeds takes dedication and effort. But those who thrive on it find it exhilarating, too, and reap fantastic fitness rewards.

## Find a Group

Having a training partner or a group of women to train with is invaluable. Having trained several times on my own for 5Ks over the years, I finally discovered a local training group in 2004 that meets once a week in the spring. Called First Strides, the group is organized by Jane Serues, fifty-six, who won the 2002 Fred LeBow Women's Running Award for her unselfish dedication to helping women find their "inner athlete."

First Strides helps women get ready for a 5K race at whatever level they feel comfortable. Some are runners increasing their speed, some are walkers who become runners over the twelve-week session, and some are walkers who learn new techniques to help them gain speed and endurance.

Now available in both Bethlehem and Allentown, Pennsylvania (and hoping to expand to a national program), First Strides is facilitated by mentors who buddy up with same-speed participants and help them through their workouts. At our first meeting, there were more than 200 women of all shapes, sizes, ages, and abilities.

My original intent was to ramp up to running. I had my son's wedding on the horizon, and I really wanted to see if running could help me drop a dress size. But the very first night, I knew running was out for me. I'd broken my ankle four months earlier; I was feeling pain from arthritis in my neck and one knee; and my back shot a couple of zingers to remind me of an old disk injury. Yikes! Who was I kidding? But rather than feeling old and discouraged, I realized that for the first time I had buddies who would stick with me for an increasingly vigorous walking program. Without the bounce of running, my ankle, neck, knees, and back would be fine. I volunteered to give walking tips to the group at every session and set my sights on powering up my stride and picking up my pace.

Participants must work out on their own during the week, but the once-a-week gathering sets the tone and pace for your commitment as you join other walkers and runners pacing themselves through a forty-five-minute workout, and pre- and post-stretch. Mentors keep tabs on the interval training for you, blowing whistles for a warm-up, easy pace, and then successive fast-paced segments, which gradually increase in duration over the twelve weeks.

Training with a group is so motivating. It's the high school track team you never had the chance to go out for. When you're alone, it's much easier to quit or slack off. But as part of the group, you gain energy from your fellow walkers, and when your motivation is flagging, someone else is on the upswing and you're carried along with it. Check with your local YMCA or recreation department to see if there is some kind of walk/run group in your area. Or start your own. You can learn more about First Strides and the possibility of creating your own group at www.firststrides.com. You may also be able to find a racewalking training group or coach through the North American Racewalking Foundation. Write to PO Box 50312, Pasadena, CA 91115-0312, or go to www.philsport.com/narf/ and look under "links."

## Choose Your Race

For your first 5K effort, I suggest you look for a run/walk. Sometimes they're called Fun Run/Walks, which suggests that their main purpose is providing a pleasant course for runners and walkers to test their skills, rather than providing a competitive racing atmosphere. Often these run/walks are created as fundraisers for a worthy cause, so the race directors want as many bodies as possible, and walkers can really help swell their ranks and their fundraising efforts. You will pay a fee to enter, usually around ten to fifteen dollars, and you'll often get a commemorative race T-shirt and goody bag when you show up. (I have so many event T-shirts I had some of them made into a quilt!) You will feel more included in such events, and there may even be prizes raffled off to the walkers after the race. There won't be any blue ribbons for walking "winners" in terms of speed, though, because of the difficulty in making sure that walkers really walk the whole way! That happens only at racewalk events. But if you're fast, you may even beat out some slow joggers.

Though you may be able to find a racewalk in your area by contacting the North American Racewalking Foundation mentioned above, you may feel somewhat overwhelmed by the details. Racewalks are judged events, meaning that judges are spread out along the course and watch to make sure the contestants maintain proper form. They check to make sure the knee is kept straight when supporting your body weight (when you bend your knee, its called creeping—think of a Groucho Marx–type walk) and to make sure you have one foot on the ground at all times (otherwise you're running). If you really enjoy racing and are competitive, you may gravitate to racewalking events in the long run, because that is where your times will really make a difference and you can win or place in events.

Look for a 5K event that's at least twelve weeks away, so you have time to train. If you're already walking regularly, you could probably easily walk a 5K and have fun doing it, and that's fine. But if you want to ramp up your fitness level, you need to gradually increase your efforts and plan your workouts to effect change in your speed and endurance.

You might want to call the race director and find out how walker-friendly the event will be. Ask if the course will stay open and the timers will stick around for the walkers. It can be kind of a bummer if you work hard at this and you feel like the race is over by the time you arrive. This happened to me several times when walking in a 10K run/walk. I remember one in which I racewalked the course, averaging thirteen-minute miles, and even though I remember passing one very slow jogger, I missed out on the post-race refreshments. The party was over! A 5K is short, and most walkers will be done in forty-five minutes if they've been training. Many runners will be completing the course in less than thirty minutes.

As you can see, it can be easy to feel like the tortoise in this kind of race setting, but remember how the fabled story goes. Slow and steady wins the race. And though you won't be beating any runners, you will be saving your body from the pounding runners are taking, you're far less likely to be injured, and you're gaining fantastic health and fitness benefits all the same.

You are a winner! So step up to the starting line and hold your head high. You'll most likely have lots of company at first. Still, I won't kid you. If you train seriously and improve your times beyond fifteen-minute miles, you may find yourself in something of a no-man's-land on the course. The runners will pull away fast, and you may find yourself leaving most of the walkers in the dust as well. Many people show up for fun run/walks just to take a pleasant stroll or a brisk walk on a road cleared of traffic. They may come with baby strollers and dogs. They will be laughing and chattering away, enjoying the weather, and the camaraderie. That's why it's great to have a training buddy. You can stick together on the walk and help each other keep up the momentum of your training times.

## Training Location

When training for your 5K, find a park, track, or trail to work out on, rather than your normal route. You want to focus on form and speed, not curbs or cars. High school tracks are a quarter-mile around, so 12 and a half laps constitutes a full 5K. It can be easy and fun to train there, but in the summer it can be hot and without any shade! I have a walking loop in the park across from my house that offers partial shade, a continuous smooth surface, and nearby bathrooms. Scout out your town for a good place to train. (You should also ask the race director about the course. Is it hilly? If so, some of your training should take place on hills.)

## Prevent Injuries

You're undertaking some rigorous training. If your shins get sore, ice them after your workout, and consider taking an over-the-counter anti-inflammatory. Be sure to stretch your calves, shins, and hamstrings religiously. Refer to the stretching and yoga sections in this book (see pages 30 and 169) to maintain flexibility and avoid injuries. If at any time during your exertions you feel light-headed, become dizzy, or have chest pain, stop your workout and check with your doctor.

## Maggie's 12-Week Workout

This is a basic pattern for a 5K training workout. It's meant to be a guideline for improving your cardiovascular and muscular conditioning and endurance. I've seen training schedules for walkers that are so complicated they've made me want to cry. This one is simple to read and simple to follow. It follows a slow progression by adding more fast walking and decreasing rest periods. It includes regular walking days (EASY), workout days (CHALLENGE), and rest days (REST!). Don't skip the rest day—it's a very important part of training! Your body needs time to recuperate and adjust to the new demands being put on it. On easy days, you'll go out and walk 30 minutes at a brisk but comfortable pace—no pushing. On these days you should feel like your walks are invigorating, not taxing.

On your challenge days, you'll be doing something called interval training, which simply means walking with a short burst of speed, then returning to a more comfortable pace, and repeating that pattern several times. This is the best way to get faster because it allows your legs, lungs, and heart to become conditioned to new demands. Always adapt the segments to your own needs by listening to your body; some days you may feel stronger and more powerful than others. Some days you may have to back off to shorter intervals of fast walking. If you're feeling really tired, having trouble sleeping, or getting grouchy, you may be overtraining. Cut back to an earlier week's schedule. But if you work with a progressive schedule, where each week you are spending a little more time in the "speed" zone and a little less time in your comfort zone, you will get faster overall.

### Planning Around Periods

Good news! If you're postmenopausal, you don't have to worry about getting your period in the middle of your 5K, or cramps the night before, or bloating or tender breasts! Yippee! If you are perimenopausal, you will have to plan for the "worst," since you may not have any idea when you are going to get your next period. Only you can decide whether it is appropriate for you to race while you have your period. Since your bleeding may be heavier than in the past, you may want to skip the event, or just walk it for fun and the experience of walking with others, without pushing the speed. A pleasant three-mile walk might even relieve cramping or premenstrual symptoms.

I want this to be a pleasant, positive experience for you. It should not feel grueling or terribly difficult. You need to adapt the following instructions to your own body, your own energy level, and your own level of enthusiasm. Interval training needn't be agonizing. If it is, you probably won't do it or you may even injure yourself. You will be experimenting with increasing your speed and then backing off, and repeating that process several times during a workout. When you speed up, you may feel your shins burning a bit, you will feel sweat on your brow and upper lip, and you should feel somewhat breathless, though still able to talk. Don't go all out, just a little bit faster than your normal brisk pace. When you ease up, don't slack to a stroll. Keep up a comfortably brisk pace that feels like a "rest" from your "pushing speed," but not so slow that it feels like you could window-shop.

It's a good idea to keep a journal as you go along and record your actual workouts and the timing of your actual intervals. Jot down how you felt before, during, and after the workout. Plan your workouts for times when your stomach is relatively empty, such as early morning, just before lunch, or just before dinner.

Determine your current per-mile pace before you start training. Use a track or trail and time your mile at a comfortably brisk pace and record it in your journal. As you progress through your training, you can test yourself periodically and watch your time for a mile decrease and your stamina increase. As you progress, walking at a faster pace will feel easier.

On your easy days, take a few minutes to practice some strengthening exercises for your shins and calves. Walk on your heels for 20 to 50 paces. Then walk normally. Follow that with walking on your tippy toes and walk another 20 to 50 paces. Repeat. This will help you on your fast days; you'll feel less burning in your shins as you speed up. The suggestions I provide for activities on your easy days are meant to stimulate your imagination. Easy days help to keep you limber, maintain a normal walking schedule, and flush out feelings of stiffness.

Begin every workout with a 5-minute warm-up and cooldown. That just means walking at a slower pace. If you feel tight in your hips, calves, or shins, take a few moments to stretch after your first 5 minutes. And always stretch at the end of your workout. (See the recommended stretches on page 30 and 169.)

# Week 1

**Monday/Wednesday/Friday:** EASY. 30-minute walk at a comfortable pace. Enjoy your surroundings! Work your shins and calves with heel walking and tiptoeing.

*Notes:* _____
_____
_____

**Tuesday/Thursday/Saturday:** CHALLENGE. Warm up for 5 minutes. Walk for 4 minutes at a comfortably brisk pace. For 1 minute, push harder. Repeat 2 additional times. Cool down for 5 minutes. Total workout time: 25 minutes, including warm-up and cooldown. Stretch.

*Notes:* _____
_____
_____

**Sunday:** REST. Or do something completely different, like kayaking. 30 minutes of yoga would be nice!

*Notes:* _____
_____
_____

# Week 2

**Monday/Wednesday/Friday:** EASY. Walk for 30 minutes. Explore new walking paths. Discover errands your can complete on foot.

*Notes:* _____
_____
_____

***Tuesday/Thursday/Saturday:*** CHALLENGE. Warm up for 5 minutes. Interval train for 18 minutes: 4 minutes comfortably brisk, 2 minutes pushing. Repeat 2 more times. Cool down for 5 minutes. Stretch. Total workout time: 28 minutes.

*Notes:* _____

_____

_____

***Sunday:*** REST. Massage your legs with oil. Take a long, hot bath or sauna. Learn some new yoga poses. Float in a pool.

*Notes:* _____

_____

_____

## Week 3

***Monday/Wednesday/Friday:*** EASY. Walk for 30 minutes at a comfortable pace. Make some walk dates with friends or family members.

*Notes:* _____

_____

_____

***Tuesday/Thursday/Saturday:*** CHALLENGE. Warm up for 5 minutes. Walk briskly for 3 minutes, and then push yourself for 2 minutes. Repeat 3 more times. Cool down for 5 minutes. Stretch. Total workout time: 30 minutes.

*Notes:* _____

_____

_____

***Sunday:*** REST. Massage your feet with oil. Relax in a hammock or lie on the floor with your feet against the wall.

*Notes:* _____

_____

_____

# Week 4

**Monday/Wednesday/Friday:** EASY. Walk for 30 minutes at a comfortable pace. Try some "waltz walking." Count "1-2-3" as you step forward, emphasizing the "1" in your mind. It's kind of fun, and you'll find you feel like you're dancing!

*Notes:* _____

_____

_____

**Tuesday/Thursday/Saturday:** CHALLENGE. Warm up for 5 minutes. Walk 3 minutes at a comfortably brisk pace, followed by 3 minutes at a little faster pace. Repeat 3 more times. Cool down for 5 minutes. Stretch. Total workout time: 34 minutes.

*Notes:* _____

_____

_____

**Sunday:** Rest. Give yourself a pedicure.

# Week 5

**Monday/Wednesday/Friday:** EASY. Walk for 30 minutes at a comfortable pace. This is a great time to walk your dog, who has been missing you! Remember to do some shin strengtheners.

*Notes:* _____

_____

_____

**Tuesday/Thursday/Saturday:** CHALLENGE. Warm up for 5 minutes. Walk 2 minutes at a comfortably brisk pace. Walk 3 minutes a little faster. Repeat 4 more times. Cool down for 5 minutes. Stretch. Total workout time: 35 minutes.

*Notes:* _____

_____

_____

*Sunday:* REST. Stretching is always a good option. Spend some time massaging your shins and calves while you watch TV.

**Note:** Your workouts are becoming more intense, and consistency is important! If you skip more than one workout in a week, you should repeat that week, rather than move forward. Your training will fall off-schedule, but you'll still be faster than when you started. You just can't skip to the next level. Your body won't be ready.

## Week 6

*Monday/Wednesday/Friday:* EASY. Walk for 20 to 30 minutes. Walk to the movies after dinner. Take a stroll to the post office. Say hello to your neighbors.

*Notes:* _____

_____

_____

*Tuesday/Thursday/Saturday:* CHALLENGE. Warm up for 5 minutes. Walk 3 minutes easy, 4 minutes hard. Repeat 3 more times. Cool down for 5 minutes. Stretch. Total workout time: 38 minutes.

*Notes:* _____

_____

_____

*Sunday:* REST. Buy some brand-new walking socks to pamper your feet. Spend some extra time stretching.

*Notes:* _____

_____

_____

# Week 7

**Monday/Wednesday/Friday:** EASY. Walk at an easy pace for 20 to 30 minutes. On one of these days, walk just a mile and time yourself. Record your time here.

*Notes:* _____

_____

_____

**Tuesday/Thursday/Saturday:** CHALLENGE. Warm up for 5 minutes. Walk 2 minutes easy, 4 minutes hard. Repeat 4 more times. Cool down for 5 minutes. Stretch. Total workout time: 40 minutes.

*Notes:* _____

_____

_____

**Sunday:** REST. Review your log. Write a few notes about how you feel about your accomplishments so far. Do a half-hour or more of yoga. Include Downward Facing Dog, Pigeon, and the runner's stretch, which focus on the hips, calves, and hamstrings.

*Notes:* _____

_____

_____

# Week 8

**Monday/Wednesday/Friday:** EASY. Walk at an easy pace for 20 to 30 minutes. Get up with the sun and watch the sunrise. Or walk after dinner with your significant other.

*Notes:* _____

_____

_____

***Tuesday/Thursday/Saturday:*** CHALLENGE. Warm up for 5 minutes. Walk for 1 minute at a comfortably brisk pace. Then walk for 4 minutes at a slightly faster pace. Repeat 5 more times. (Basically, you're taking 1-minute rest breaks throughout the workout.) Cool down for 5 minutes. Stretch. Total workout time: 40 minutes.

*Notes:* _____

_____

_____

***Sunday:*** REST. Focus on your eating habits today. Search for some healthy treat recipes to replace any store-bought sweet you succumb to after a workout.

*Notes:* _____

_____

_____

## Week 9

***Monday/Wednesday/Friday:*** EASY. Walk for 20 to 30 minutes at a comfortable pace. Make some walking dates with friends and catch up with them while you stride.

*Notes:* _____

_____

_____

***Tuesday/Thursday/Saturday:*** CHALLENGE. Warm up for 5 minutes. Walk at a comfortable pace for 1 minute, then walk a little faster for 5 minutes. Repeat 5 more times. Cool down for 5 minutes. Stretch. Total workout time: 46 minutes.

*Notes:* _____

_____

_____

**Sunday:** REST. Massage your feet today with some nice foot cream with peppermint in it. Do some yoga stretches, and end with your feet elevated on the seat of a chair.

*Notes:*

---

## Week 10

**Monday/Wednesday/Friday:** EASY. Walk at an easy pace for 20 to 30 minutes. Feel free to break up your walk into 10-minute segments throughout your day.

*Notes:*

---

**Tuesday/Thursday/Saturday:** CHALLENGE. You're getting close to your event and finding a consistent pace for the entire 5K. Warm up for 5 minutes. Walk 1 minute at a comfortably brisk pace. Walk 7 minutes at a faster pace. Repeat 4 more times. Cool down for 5 minutes. Stretch. Total workout time: 50 minutes.

*Notes:*

---

**Sunday:** REST. Extra stretching will help keep the kinks out of your calves, hamstrings, and hips. Take a warm bath or shower and spend 30 to 60 minutes in luxurious yoga stretches.

*Notes:*

---

# Week 11

**Monday/Wednesday/Friday:** EASY. Your workouts are getting more intense on your alternate days. If you feel overly tired or sore, take an extra rest day. Otherwise, walk at a comfortable pace for 20 to 30 minutes.

*Notes:* _____

_____

_____

**Tuesday/Thursday/Saturday:** CHALLENGE. You're an athlete! How do you feel? Warm up for 5 minutes. Stretch your calves, shins, and hamstrings. Walk for 1 minute at a comfortably brisk pace. Then walk a little faster for 9 minutes. Repeat 3 more times. Cool down for 5 minutes. Stretch. Total workout time: 50 minutes. Pat yourself on the back!

*Notes:* _____

_____

_____

**Sunday:** Rest! Spend some time visualizing your race. If you can, go out and drive the course to become familiar with it. See yourself walking strong and completing the course feeling invigorated!

*Notes:* _____

_____

_____

# Week 12

**You made it! Congratulations!**
**Monday/Wednesday/Friday:** EASY. Instead of walking, take the time to stretch luxuriously each of these days. (You can warm up for the stretching by walking for 5 minutes, even if it's simply in place, inside your house.) You're resting up for the big day.

*Notes:* _____

_____

_____

**Tuesday/Thursday:** CHALLENGE. Focus on pacing yourself. Try counting the number of steps you take for 1 minute. This can help you pace yourself during the race. It's so easy to slow down when you're distracted! Warm up for 5 minutes. (Imagine this is your pre-race warm-up.) Then begin walking at a pace you feel you can sustain for 45 minutes. (Of course, you will ebb and flow some. But strive for consistency.) Cool down for 5 minutes. Stretch. Total walking time: 55 minutes. (Most likely, you'll be walking farther than a 5K by now!)

*Notes:* _____

_____

_____

**Saturday:** Race Day! The actual race should feel like a breeze! Your per-mile time may be 15 minutes or faster, so your total walking time for the 5K may be 45 minutes or less. Enjoy the race. Feel your strength, energy, and vitality! Don't overdo or push too hard!

*Notes:* _____

_____

_____

## Race Day!

If you've completed this training with any consistency, you should feel very proud of your efforts. You've probably shaved several minutes off your pace, and you're feeling wonderful about it. Make this a fun day. Celebrate your achievement!

Eat a light breakfast, like oatmeal and fruit, and drink some water so you're hydrated when you get to the race area. Don't drink coffee or tea since they tend to make you have to go to the bathroom! Dress in layers if you need to stay warm, but toss those extra layers in your car before the race starts. Wear a hat or visor and sunglasses on sunny days so you don't have to drop your head to avoid glare.

Show up early so you can find a good parking spot, register, and get yourself mentally and physically ready. Once you're registered (you may get a number and an event T-shirt), take some time to warm up by walking briskly for about ten minutes. Stretch your calves, shins, hips, and hamstrings. Locate the bathrooms; you'll probably feel the need to go before the race.

Runners will be starting first, so that walkers won't be mowed down by them on course. Then the event coordinator will call the walkers to the starting line. Don't worry about being out in front. A shot may be fired, or a bell rung, or someone may just say, "On your mark, get set, go!" Don't start out too fast! Just find your pace and glide along. Enjoy!

At the finish line, you'll pass the timer. Remember to look for your time! There may not be anyone recording the times of walkers, since there aren't prizes based on time. There will probably be some flags to direct you to the "chute" where the finish line and timing device is. You're done! But don't stop now. Keep walking to cool down. Then grab some water (the race coordinators often make water and post-race snacks available). Layer up again if it's cold. You'll want to stick around for any prizes that may be raffled off. Enjoy the spirit and camaraderie of the event. And keep an eye out for future training partners!

# Walk with Your Best Friend: Dogs as Walking Partners

**Try this program if**

- you and/or your dog are overweight and/or out of shape;
- you've wanted a dog for a long time, and now that your kids are grown, you're finally ready to care for one;
- you realize the benefit of having a walking partner, but you don't want one you'll have to talk to all the time;
- you feel vulnerable walking alone.

**What you'll need:** A breed of dog that loves the outdoors and that you can handle. Ask your vet whether the dog you have is a good candidate for a walking program. If you don't have a dog, but have been planning a purchase or adoption, call a local vet and see what kind of dog she recommends for your climate. Pug-faced dogs don't make good walking companions. Rottweilers and other large dogs may overpower you on the road unless they're trained to heel.

## Walking Your Dog, Walking You

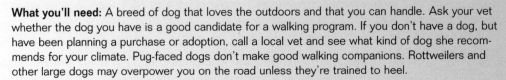

According to the Humane Society, there are about 65 million "owned" dogs in the United States. Well over a third of U.S. households have at least one dog. Hold that figure in mind and consider the fact that there are only about 10 million women fitness walking (which means walking at least three days a week). While 23 million women and 14 million men say they walk for recreation at least once a week, that still leaves almost half the U.S. dog population out of luck—even if we were to surmise that all those walkers are taking their dogs with them, which I assure you they are not.

Because of those statistics, I would never say that owning a dog is a sure-fire way to enhance your chances of sustaining a walking regimen. And I would never recommend that a person get a dog because they believe having one will force them to exercise. If that were true, the American Sports Data Superstudy would find far more walkers out there than they do now!

I've known many people who have very close relationships with their pets. But I've also known plenty who get a dog who eventually becomes more like a moveable piece of furniture that requires daily doses of protein. They feed him and step over him, but don't give him much attention, much less take him for walks. Taking your dog for regular walks can give both of you a new leash on life—and you may be surprised at how much more interesting and alive your dog seems to you as you get to know each other this way.

The two of you could improve your health, maybe lose some weight—your dog may fare better than you, since he can't drive to Dunkin' Donuts on a whim—and get a *whole lot more love and satisfaction from your relationship!*

I grew up in a dog family. We usually had three at once, all shapes and sizes. And I have to admit, rarely did anyone but my mother walk those dogs. We didn't have a fenced-in yard, and our dogs were never left out unattended. So walking was the only way they got to take care of business. My mother would walk them all at once, usually with a cigarette in hand. She would meander to the end of the block and back—not exactly what I'd call exercise.

It wasn't until my midthirties that I got a dog that became a walking buddy. (Ironically, my mother adopted him for me.) His name was Petey, and he was part Japanese Chin, but sturdier than the pure breeds. He lived with me for 17 years, and he loved to walk and did well even though he had a puglike face, though on hot days he'd sometimes lie down in a shady spot and refuse to move any farther. He was only about 15 pounds, and it was easy to take him in the car to my favorite walking trails. I had adopted a golden retriever once but ended up giving him away. He wanted to run, not walk, and I didn't have the time, energy, or desire to give him the kind of exercise he really needed.

Now I have a cockapoo (a combination of cocker spaniel and poodle) named Puppy. She was my mother's last dog, and my mom was so forgetful that Puppy was the only name she could remember. When she died of Alzheimer's three years after getting her, Puppy came home with me. Puppy is a wonderful walking partner and is the first dog I have ever owned that I can let off lead to walk beside me—though I do this only in parks or on the canal towpath. I find that to be the most pleasurable way of walking with a dog, and I'd always been jealous of people who had dogs that would stick by them that way. I allow Puppy a certain latitude to look into things she's interested in while I keep walking. She lags behind for a moment from time to time, then runs to catch up with me. We're both having a great time! Though she's small, she can hike or walk for four or five miles.

Over the years, I've written several stories about walking with your dog and advised people to take their dogs to obedience classes so that walking is more of a pleasure than a pain. I still recommend this, but I also know that most people never do it. They don't have enough time, money, or patience. So this time, my advice is going to be very practical; I'm going to assume that your dog has always been something of a nit-wit on a walk and that it's up to you to make the experience as pleasurable for both of you as possible. If your dog isn't trained to heel, you need the appropriate collar and leash to make the best of it.

Here are my suggestions for beginning a walking program together:

- Take your dog to the vet (and yourself to the doctor) to make sure that you can start walking together without adversely affecting your dog's or your own health.

- Use a harness, rather than a collar. If your dog has not been taught to heel and is going to be pulling at times, any collar will be choking him to some degree. A harness is far more comfortable. I've also considered it much safer when walking places where the dog might accidentally slip off a ledge or boardwalk. You can haul a dog up relatively safely in a harness, but you'll hang him by his collar!

- If you have a big, strong, untrained dog that pulls your arm halfway out of its socket while the two of you are walking down the street, get a special harness, available in pet stores, that will keep him from doing so. I've tried the Sporn Dog Harness with success. (My son's male pit bull immediately stopped pulling when wearing it.) It puts pressure on an area behind the front legs, rather than on the neck. (Please, don't use spiked collars!) It's amazing to witness. The dog isn't in pain, but just senses immediately that he can't pull. It's ASPCA approved and well worth the moderate price.

- Buy a retractable leash: This allows you to swing your arms back and forth while you walk, without pulling your dog (who's probably not heeling, but out in front of you forging ahead) over backwards. They come in various sizes.

- Try to get your dog to defecate at home, not on the trail or in a neighbor's yard. If you haven't gotten that far, then always carry a bag to clean up after your pet. This is just common courtesy and should be done out of concern for public health. I keep plastic grocery bags in a cloth dispenser by my back door. I grab a leash, then a bag.

- Be aware that your dog's paws are not indestructible! If it's too hot for you to walk on blacktop barefoot, it's not good for your dog either! And if you're out in snow or ice, make sure your dog's feet aren't getting clogged with anything frozen or the chemicals people use to melt ice. (Protective booties are available, too.) While sidewalks help keep your dog's nails trimmed, take him on softer, natural dirt paths and grass, too.

- Apply flea and tick medication regularly. Once you start walking your dog, you expose him to the possibility of infestation. Your house or yard may be flea free, but a neighbor's may not. (When I lived in downtown Allentown, I once walked around the block in the fall, kicking through fallen leaves. When I got home, there were lots of fleas clinging to my pale-colored sweatpants.) I use the highly recommended Frontline once a month. If a flea or tick bites an animal that has been treated with Frontline, the bug will die. I wish they had something like that for people to use, so we could all avoid Lyme disease!

- If you're walking long enough or in temperatures where you might want a drink of water, bring something along to give your dog a drink, too. I have a soft, foldable cloth bowl. Sometimes your dog will drink from your cupped hand, but you can waste a lot of water that way!

- Work up your mileage gradually. If your dog is very overweight, it may take a while before she can go any real distance with you. Take her around the block and drop her off if she seems tired or is panting too heavily. Then finish your walk on your own.

- Always have something in your car to wipe off your dog's paws if you drive her to a trail. A dog's fur and paws can be a magnet for dirt and gravel. I protect the car seat with the towel I bring to clean off my dog's paws.

- Beware of walking in unfamiliar neighborhoods with your dog. This is a problem for me, living in the country. A few people do have large dogs unattended on their properties. A small dog like mine that tends to yip a lot can get a normally calm dog really riled up. And some dogs are just nasty when it comes to protecting their turf. I never want to have to intervene in a dogfight. I walk Puppy only where I know we won't be bothered.

Dog parks are becoming more popular. They're places specifically created and maintained for dogs to get some exercise and play with other dogs. I first saw one in New York City and thought, "What fun!" But as more and more suburban community parks become off-limits to dogs, dog parks are cropping up in suburban areas, too. If you decide to use a dog park, just make sure you get exercise, too! Don't drive there—or at least don't drive all the way there. Park at least a mile away and walk your dog to playtime.

I think I'll always have a dog. For me, they help make a house a home. And they do make great walking buddies. They never want to read the Sunday paper or watch a football game instead. You glance at the leash and they're at the door, ready and willing. They help lower your blood pressure, boost your mood, and help you feel safe at night. (Even if they wouldn't or couldn't hurt a flea.)

### Maggie Loves Cockapoos

Here's why I love poodles and cockapoos:
- they are very, very smart and easily trainable
- they don't shed. (No kidding!)
- they have little dander (they are nonallergenic)
- they love to walk and are very loyal dogs
- they come in all sizes
- they can be clipped in summer to endure the heat
- they can be shaggy in winter to help tolerate the cold
- they are beautiful, sturdy, and live a long time.

## The Walk-Your-Dog Beginner Program

Use this space to record your walks both alone and with your dog. Your aim is for a minimum of 30 minutes a day of brisk walking, based on the surgeon general's recommendations for health. But in the beginning, you may find it optimal for both you and your dog to split your walk into three 10-minute segments.

You may want to let your dog run in your yard, if possible, to release pent-up energy before starting your walk together. He may be calmer and easier to handle on a leash afterwards.

## Veterinary Checkup Date:

Results/Notes: _____

_____

_____

_____

_____

## Flea and Tick Application:

Date: _____

Date: _____

Date: _____

Date: _____

| | Minutes/Miles | Weather/Temperature | Terrain | Notes |
|---|---|---|---|---|
| | | | | |
| **Monday** | | | | |
| | | | | |
| **Tuesday** | | | | |
| | | | | |
| **Wednesday** | | | | |
| | | | | |
| **Thursday** | | | | |
| | | | | |
| **Friday** | | | | |
| | | | | |
| **Saturday** | | | | |
| | | | | |
| **Sunday** | | | | |
| | | | | |

# Walk to the Beat: Music as Motivator

**Try this program if you**
- love music but never seem to find the time to listen anymore;
- want to pick up your pace almost effortlessly;
- enjoy getting a natural "high" while walking;
- tend to take shorter walks than you'd like;
- walk mostly on a treadmill;
- want to boost your brainpower while walking;
- need to be distracted while you walk, perhaps because you get bored easily.

**What you'll need:** A portable CD or cassette player, appropriate music or walking programs, batteries.

*"Dancers need music, but walkers are their own music."*

—*W.A. Mathieu,* The Listening Book

Music is a powerful motivator. It activates our souls and our cells. We know that the vibrations we call music can aid healing and boost our brainpower. Studies have shown that listening to Mozart before an exam helps students improve test scores. You probably don't need a study to tell you that when you listen to music while exercising, you tend to exercise harder and longer than without music. You're focusing on the feelings evoked by the music, not on your breathing or your sore knee. The first time I put on a pair of headphones and headed out for a walk, I was astounded at how the sense of being in the center of the music while walking could give me such a powerful expansion of energy and ebullience. It's hard not to break into whirls, twirls, and leaps, like a member of a Broadway musical. (In fact, on a secluded walk, I have done just that.)

However, there is a cautionary note here: Play the music too loud, and you can damage your hearing. In fact, listening to headphones while you exercise vigorously can even make your ears more vulnerable. It's a good idea to keep your volume at half the maximum. You should be able to carry on a conversation even with your headphones on. An hour a day is probably okay, unless you're already exposed to loud noise during your day.

There is also the risk of being attacked or robbed while absorbed in your music. Walking with a buddy can help. But you have to use your own judgment as to whether an area is safe for walking with music. If you're at all concerned about your safety, either from traffic, strangers, or stray dogs, then it's best to leave your headphones at home.

That's why I suggest two ways to add music to your walking workouts: the electronic way of listening to CDs and cassettes, and the natural way of making your own music or listening to the natural music around you.

Years ago, a friend recommended I read *The Listening Book: Discovering Your Own Music*, by musician, composer, and teacher W. A. Mathieu. Mathieu points out that walking tempo is basic to all music because it's basic to all people; it's a central, internal tempo. He suggests games to play when walking, games that are enjoyable simply for their own sake, that play with tempo. For instance, normally we walk with a steady, rhythmic gait, where one foot is slightly more dominant. We walk *Left*, right, *Left*, right, or *Right*, left, *Right*, left, with our dominant foot corresponding to our dominant hand. Some have suggested that this rhythmic left-right tempo and action of our arms and legs is what makes walking so soothing and stokes our creativity. But try mixing up that rhythm for a moment. Start out by counting "One, two, One, two" as your feet hit the ground. Then switch to this accented rhythm: "*One*, two, three, *One*, two, three, *One*, two three." Each time you think "One," you'll be stepping forward with a different foot. This is the rhythm of the waltz, and walking this way will make you feel like you're dancing down the street, whether you have music or not. Try it— you'll be fascinated by its effect. You're waltz-walking! If you know a waltz tune, hum along!

You can also sing or whistle when you walk. You don't have to be loud, but hopefully you have places to walk where few people (if anyone) can hear you and make you feel self-conscious. (This is a great test of lung power, too.) I have always lamented the fact that our society for the most part leaves music-making to professionals, and that singing and playing musical instruments is not a part of our everyday life, as it has been in earlier cultures. Long before television kept us entertained, families sang together or played musical instruments to pass the time. When I was a kid and went walking and hiking with friends, we invariably broke out into a chorus of "The Happy Wanderer." When climbing the Alps in Switzerland, someone inevitably starts singing, "The hills are alive…with the sound of music…"

and the group joins in. But for the most part, we're embarrassed to sing spontaneously in front of others, and group singing is seldom encountered in day-to-day life or family life. And I believe we are greatly impoverished by that loss.

In *The Listening Book*, Mathieu talks about someday wanting to be in a walking choir. "We march down farming roads and through bedroom communities, stomp across malls and over bridges and tramp through industrial parks.... We'll sing a little Beach Boys and Bach and a lot of gospel...just throats and feet and banners blowing." I would want to be in that choir!

Now, I know you're not going to walk around the block in your neighborhood belting out "Satisfaction" by the Rolling Stones (though that would be a great way to disperse negative energy—*"I can't get no...duh duh daaaa...satisfaction! "*). But try a little waltz-walking and humming. And if you find a private place to walk, sing away. I like to sing childhood songs with simple melodies or things I learned in various school choirs, like "You'll Never Walk Alone." If you have young grandchildren in tow, I bet they'll gladly sing with you!

Another way to bring "music" into your walk is simply to listen intently to all that's going on around you. Paying attention to sounds will help you turn off your incessant mental chatter. Attention, says Eckhart Tolle in *Stillness Speaks,* is consciousness itself, and through attention, we gain wisdom. You may find early morning walks are a wonderful time to listen to bird songs. When I'm feeling lonely, I love walking around a nearby park when the summer playground is open. The sounds of children chattering, calling, and laughing float around the track I walk on, and I find that uplifting and somehow consoling. This kind of listening is an active, not a passive, process. If you don't pay attention, the sounds literally seem to disappear as you become preoccupied with your own thoughts.

## Walkman Magic

Bringing music on a walk with you is truly a marvel of modern times. When I was a kid, I occasionally walked with a transistor radio plugged into one ear. (Remember those days?) But of course that didn't compare to the sounds of stereo headphones and digital recordings. Choosing music to walk with is purely a matter of taste and a feeling for tempo. While some people love marches, others love rock 'n roll. But there is so much out there that will work, you need only experiment to find what works for you.

One of my most memorable walks of all time was taken with a friend in the middle of a snow fall. I was listening to *Silk Road* by Kitaro, which is full of glistening, crystalline sounds. We walked through thickets and woods filling up with big, wet, heavy snowflakes that coated every branch, creating a magical, wonderland effect. After about forty-five minutes of being completely absorbed in the interplay between the music and the seemingly soundless winter scenery, we emerged from the woods as though from another world. After twenty years, I still marvel at the power and perfection of that walk. This is a different kind of walk with music. The effect is one of awe and connection to nature, rather than a focus on pace. The music seems to amplify the natural world, not displace it. For this kind of walk with music, I recommend works by composer and recording artist Steve Halperin, who wrote *Sound Health*. Recordings such as "Dawn," "Comfort Zone," and "Spectrum Suite" are designed to create a relaxed, alert state of mind and seem to complement the sights I see on a nature walk, rather than compete with them. But there are many options in the music world to explore.

Of course, there are cassettes and CDs made for walkers that are specifically paced for people walking between a twenty- and fifteen-minute-per-mile pace, or even faster. They sometimes have coaching on form and include encouraging words. I've produced two of these myself, called *Power Up Your Stride*, which uses marches, and *Swing Your Way to Weight Loss*, which uses big band, swing, and show tunes. (Go to **www.walkforallseasons.com** for more information.) These can be great when you want to increase your speed or familiarize yourself with a specific pace and get your heart rate into your target range. Plus, often you'll be told how long you've been walking, and how far. And some programs, like mine, will take you through a stretching routine as well.

I've found that walking programs set to music tend to grow on you as you use them. The first day, you're very curious and paying attention to the coaching. But by midweek, you're becoming familiar with the voice and the music, and they start to feel like real partners on your walk. And it's as though your body responds instantly to the lead song or the first words of welcome from the coach. You find yourself humming along, anticipating the next song, and your body anticipates the increases in pacing or the interval training. So I suggest using recorded walking program for at least a week at a time.

If you walk on a treadmill most of the time or if you head inside during freezing or steaming-hot weather, music may be the only thing that keeps you sane. I find treadmills a sorry alternative to walking out of doors, but I will use them when it feels like I'm freezing my face off outside. If your health club plays music, I suggest you still consider bringing your own. Most of the time, I find piped-in music obnoxious, not my taste, or low quality.

You can find paced walking recordings online at The Walkers Warehouse (www.walkerswarehouse.com) or Collage Video (www.collagevideo.com). Collage also has a paper catalog, available by calling the following toll-free number (in the United States and Canada only): (800) 819-7111. Sometimes department stores like K-mart or Walmart may carry them, but these stores won't have nearly the selection that's available online or through catalogs.

If you don't already have one, you'll need a portable CD player or cassette player. But I still prefer cassette players as they don't skip, and a lot of my music collection is cassette based.

Also, the new technology of iPods and MP3 players are ideal companions for a walker, because of their versatility. Being able to download and arrange your favorite songs allows you to pick the perfect tunes for your walks. Choose songs that match your mood and walking rythms. It's like having your own personal movie soundtrack!

I usually just slip my player into a pocket while I walk, but I also have a carrier case made out of stretchy neoprene that wraps around my waist. That's actually the best way to carry a walkman, but sometimes I just get lazy. I bring extra batteries because it's *really* frustrating to head out for a brisk walk and have the music start slowing down halfway through.

## Getting Started

Spend a Sunday afternoon sorting through your available music collection. If you're like me, you have plenty of good music lying around in cabinets, in boxes, and under the bed that you haven't listened to in years. You might feel like you're getting ready for a reunion of sorts. Music will evoke old memories in a powerful way, so be aware. You may not want to choose an album from the '60s that you played every day during a painful breakup or some other dramatic time in your life.

Another option is to create your own walking music album by downloading music from the Internet and onto an MP3 player or iPod. Don't know how to do that? Ask your kids (or somebody else's kids). My son has created several albums for me full of songs I love.

You may find that sorting through your music collection puts you in a partying mood. Great! Have a party. Kick off your "Walk to the Beat" program with some popcorn and iced tea and listen to great tunes with your friends. Maybe you can recruit somebody to walk with you. You may both be in your private music worlds once you put your headphones on, but it's still very helpful to have a buddy to meet for exercise, and you're always safer when walking in a pair.

If you want to get some coaching in, search the catalogs above and order something. If you're just getting back into exercise, stick with beginner paces, like twenty minutes per mile. But if you've been walking for several months or more and you're trying to rev up your pace for weight loss or more energy, look for faster paces. A fifteen-minute-per-mile pace is quite brisk for most people, but there are faster programs for the winged-footed and athletic walker.

I suggest making yourself a little "altar" for daily exercise. Find a place to put your player, music, walking shoes, and batteries every time you come in from a walk. Make it someplace plainly visible, to serve as a pleasant reminder. Or keep your stash in your car, if you do your walking away from home. Stow extra pairs of socks as well as a zip-lock baggie to store your sweaty socks so your car doesn't smell like a locker room. If your walking shoes smell, try dumping a little baking soda in them.

If there's an album you've been meaning to buy, or an artist you want to catch up with, indulge now. Or just spend an hour browsing through the music collections in a store. Have you seen a great musical in the last few years and would like to relive it? Buy the soundtrack. (I went to see Mamma Mia on Broadway last year, with music by ABBA—a great choice for walking music!)

## The Walk to the Beat Program

The way you approach this program depends entirely upon your needs and desires. If you're looking for motivation and ways to stay enthused or entertained while walking, then just keep a record of how it goes. For example, list the albums you listened to and how long and/or how far you walked. Record your feelings at the end of the walk. Then you can begin to evaluate how effective music is in motivating you. Do you walk more often, for longer periods of time? Are you walking more briskly with music and enjoying it more?

If you're using walking music that's designed to help you pick up the pace, or interval train, you may want to alternate hard days with easier days until the faster pace feels comfortable.

In addition, I suggest some "rest" days, when you walk without headphones and spend time listening to nature, humming, or chanting. Or you might try some waltz-walking on these days.

### Pick the Perfect Pace

My friends James and Karen Sundquist, of Last Generations Artists, Inc., musicians, teachers, and the producers of my audiotapes, understand perfectly which musical styles will keep you walking at specific speeds. There are variations in how these styles are performed, but the following list is a great starting point for weeding through your collection or taking with you to the music store. The list is based on the beats per minute (bpm) of the music, which relates to how many steps per minute you will take when listening to these musical styles:

- 100 bpm (two mph or a thirty-minute mile): classical, bolero, slow waltzes, blues, reggae, rumba, samba, hip-hop
- 120 bpm (three mph or a twenty-minute mile): march, rock, mainstream pop, disco, soul, ragtime, Broadway show tunes, country, slow fox-trot, tango, big band
- 140 bpm (four mph or a fifteen-minute mile): techno pop, big band, classical, jazz, square dance, polka
- 170 bpm (five mph or a twelve-minute mile): Dixieland, boogie-woogie, jazz, national jive, classical, Viennese waltz, bluegrass, jungle (drum and bass)

| WEEK 1 | Music | Time/ Distance | Tempo or Pace | Notes |
|---|---|---|---|---|
| | | | | |
| Monday | | | | |
| | | | | |
| Tuesday | | | | |
| | | | | |
| Wednesday | | | | |
| | | | | |
| Thursday | | | | |
| | | | | |
| Friday | | | | |
| | | | | |
| Saturday | | | | |
| | | | | |
| Sunday | | | | |
| | | | | |

| WEEK 2 | Music | Time/Distance | Tempo or Pace | Notes |
|---|---|---|---|---|
| | | | | |
| **Monday** | | | | |
| | | | | |
| **Tuesday** | | | | |
| | | | | |
| **Wednesday** | | | | |
| | | | | |
| **Thursday** | | | | |
| | | | | |
| **Friday** | | | | |
| | | | | |
| **Saturday** | | | | |
| | | | | |
| **Sunday** | | | | |
| | | | | |

| WEEK 3 | Music | Time/ Distance | Tempo or Pace | Notes |
|--------|-------|----------------|---------------|-------|
| Monday | | | | |
| Tuesday | | | | |
| Wednesday | | | | |
| Thursday | | | | |
| Friday | | | | |
| Saturday | | | | |
| Sunday | | | | |

| WEEK 4 | Music | Time/Distance | Tempo or Pace | Notes |
|---|---|---|---|---|
| **Monday** | | | | |
| | | | | |
| **Tuesday** | | | | |
| | | | | |
| **Wednesday** | | | | |
| | | | | |
| **Thursday** | | | | |
| | | | | |
| **Friday** | | | | |
| | | | | |
| **Saturday** | | | | |
| | | | | |
| **Sunday** | | | | |
| | | | | |

*Walk Your Way Through Menopause*

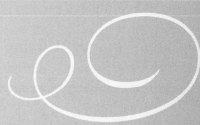

## PROGRAM 9

# *Winter or Summer Indoors*

**Try this program when**

- it's too hot or too cold to walk outside;
- your outdoor allergies flair up and you don't like to medicate;
- you're in charge of the grandkids (or you're still raising your own children), and you can't leave the house;
- your neighborhood is not a pleasant or safe place to walk alone;
- you're self-conscious about exercising in public (though I know you'll get over it!).

**What you'll need:** A TV and VCR or DVD player, access to a large indoor shopping mall, a motorized treadmill or access to one, or other decent piece of aerobic equipment (optional)

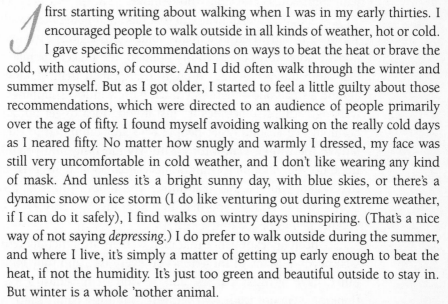

*I* first starting writing about walking when I was in my early thirties. I encouraged people to walk outside in all kinds of weather, hot or cold. I gave specific recommendations on ways to beat the heat or brave the cold, with cautions, of course. And I did often walk through the winter and summer myself. But as I got older, I started to feel a little guilty about those recommendations, which were directed to an audience of people primarily over the age of fifty. I found myself avoiding walking on the really cold days as I neared fifty. No matter how snugly and warmly I dressed, my face was still very uncomfortable in cold weather, and I don't like wearing any kind of mask. And unless it's a bright sunny day, with blue skies, or there's a dynamic snow or ice storm (I do like venturing out during extreme weather, if I can do it safely), I find walks on wintry days uninspiring. (That's a nice way of not saying *depressing*.) I do prefer to walk outside during the summer, and where I live, it's simply a matter of getting up early enough to beat the heat, if not the humidity. It's just too green and beautiful outside to stay in. But winter is a whole 'nother animal.

So you've come to this section of the book because it's hot or cold and you don't want to go outside. I'm going to give you some very specific instructions for keeping a walking-based exercise program going for the months that you go into "hibernation," but I encourage you to add anything else to the pot that attracts you. Ask other people you know who obviously stay in shape what *they* do. Maybe they take belly-dancing lessons or go country line dancing three nights a week. Or maybe they play a hot game of

121

table tennis. (This is a great indoor game I love to play, too. I have a table in my basement.) Experiment, explore, push yourself a little to try new things. You'll meet new people and find new strengths and ways to play. And that helps keep you young in body, mind, and spirit!

## Indoor Walking Solutions

For now, I'm going to recommend a regimen of indoor walking. You can accomplish it several ways, and I suggest you use all three if you can, just to keep from getting bored or isolated.

First, get some videos or DVDs so you can work out in front of your TV. Many exercise videos, especially ones geared to walking, are simple enough that you're not straining your brain, but they are lively enough and have enough variety to keep you engaged. Leslie Sansone has some good ones, and I also like *Kathy Smith's Fat-Burning Workout*, which is basically walking with some squats and upper-body moves to keep your heart rate pumping.

Second, find a mall near you that has an ongoing mall-walking program. You may be surprised how many malls have legions of walkers pacing the floors before stores open. In my opinion, the bigger the mall the better. It's just more fun wandering through a large mall than making a lot of laps around a small one—there's so much more window shopping! I suggest mall walking because sometimes it's just a good idea to get out and really walk again and be around other people who are committed to exercise, particularly in the winter. Plan it for a Saturday morning, and you'll be all pepped up to do your shopping errands afterwards. Some malls even have an incentive system you can join that allows you to win prizes or discounts at the stores. And of course, you may find a buddy. You may even find a mate, if you happen to be looking for one!

It's been my experience that mall walkers are generally retirement age or well beyond. Many of these folks go every day, and they look out for each other, have birthday parties, and go out for breakfast a lot. You may be thinking, "I'm not ready for that, yet!" But it is a handy place to walk in bad weather; there are water fountains, bathrooms, and security guards. Striding past the retirees, you may feel young and lively! But you may also find there are plenty of women your age who are taking advantage of the air-conditioned comfort. People who have had heart attacks and have been told by their doctors to walk every day often resort to malls because heat or cold stresses their cardiovascular system too much.

Third, find a treadmill. I'm not saying to invest in one, necessarily. I know how many of them end up collecting dust in someone's basement. But that doesn't mean yours automatically will. Still, they are a big investment. A decent one is going to cost at least $600, and most are a lot more. (Nonmotorized treadmills are very difficult to walk on, and I would rule them out altogether.) Look in the classifieds for used ones. Or join a gym where you can use one. This year I found a club that I can join one month at a time. I pay a higher monthly price, about $60 per month as opposed to $40, but that works for me. Actually, I do have a treadmill in my basement, but I much prefer going to the club with my friend who walks on the treadmill next to me.

Another, less expensive option is to find a stationary bicycle. (I prefer indoor walking to indoor biking, which seems to concentrate so much of the effort on a couple of muscles in your thighs, but you should choose whichever most motivates you.) Put whatever machine you get in front of the TV and hop on during the news or your favorite program. Pop in a movie and tell yourself you can watch it only as long as you're exercising. I love watching old family videos when I'm treadmilling.

I also enjoy just listening to music and working on my posture and stride (a mirror helps). I've been known to sing on the treadmill, too, though I usually reserve that treat for an empty house.

If you don't have the resources to buy a piece of equipment or join a gym, then find some stairs. They could be in your own house, at your workplace, or in an indoor stadium at a local college. (I've joined my daughter-in-law at the local high school for an indoor workout that includes several loops of going down three flights of stairs, walking to the end of a hall, and then climbing back up three flights!) Climbing stairs is a great workout for your heart and lungs and your legs and butt. Just build up gradually, increasing the number of steps and the speed or intensity so that you always feel invigorated, rather than exhausted, after a step workout.

I also suggest taking a class of some sort when the weather outside is frightful (either too hot or too cold). Last winter I took a series of tap lessons. I suggest yoga, tap, belly dancing, country line dancing, tai chi, kickboxing, Pilates—anything that is fun and keeps reminding you that you're a person who loves to be active!

These are all great options for keeping yourself healthy and fit when outdoor conditions have you holed up. Below is a chart with a suggested program mapped out for you. It's based on the idea of maintaining the surgeon general's recommendation of 30 minutes a day of moderately intense exercise, most days of the week. Adapt it to your own needs and circumstances. Use the blank chart to create your own, individualized chart. Then keep notes on how well you meet your weekly goals.

*Monday:* Indoor walking video, 30 to 60 minutes (before breakfast or before dinner—maybe while something's cooking)

*Tuesday:* Walk on your treadmill or pedal your stationary bike during the morning or evening news.

*Wednesday*: Indoor walking video, 30 minutes

*Thursday:* Go to an evening dance, yoga, aerobics, tai chi—whatever—class

*Friday:* Indoor walking video, 30 minutes

*Saturday:* Go to the mall for an early morning walking workout, then shopping. Bring a buddy if possible, and keep each other away from the cinnamon buns, giant pretzels, and ice cream cones! Opt for a frozen fruit bar or a McDonald's fresh fruit and yogurt cup.

*Sunday:* Take a day off or bundle up and brave the cold with someone you love. If it's hot, take a romantic walk after it gets dark. Or find a place to go swimming together.

*Note:* On any one of these days, even a few minutes of yoga stretches will feel great!

Now create your own schedule based on your time and resources. To me, lots of variety is always important, especially with indoor programs because I can get bored easily. But if you love working with videos, for instance, then do them as often as you like. It's your program. Do what works for you.

| | Location or Treadmill | Speed | How did I feel? |
|---|---|---|---|
| **Monday** | | | |
| | | | |
| **Tuesday** | | | |
| | | | |
| **Wednesday** | | | |
| | | | |
| **Thursday** | | | |
| | | | |
| **Friday** | | | |
| | | | |
| **Saturday** | | | |
| | | | |
| **Sunday** | | | |
| | | | |

# Stalking Historic Landmarks

**Try this program if you**
- feel like you're getting older, but not better;
- search your face for wrinkles or sagging jowls every morning;
- need intellectual stimulation to keep your walks interesting or to exercise your brain;
- have always been drawn to or interested in old houses and historic buildings but don't know what you're looking at;
- would like to learn more about the history of your town or area, but you've never found the time.

**What you'll need:** A library card, curiosity about history, neighborhoods you can explore, this quick guide to architectural styles, a map of your town or surrounding towns. A step counter for gauging how far you walk will come in handy; as you explore, your mind won't be on distance or time.

Which one of us has not stood in front of the mirror examining our deepening laugh lines, sagging jowls, or dimples turning into furrows? For many women, the relentless process of aging can undermine feelings of self-worth and self-esteem as we realize that despite healthful behaviors or miracle creams and cleansers, *we ain't getting any younger.* When I was turning forty, I remember having many conversations with friends about how we felt as if we were becoming invisible. There was a definite sense that when we entered a room, heads no longer turned our way. Depending on how much your sense of self was derived from your figure or your face, the postmenopausal years can seem like you're sliding down an increasingly slippery slope.

The following walking program is not about how to look younger, taller, or slimmer. Still, I can tell you that recent research suggests that regular exercisers do have fewer wrinkles. (And that's not just right after a walk, when your skin is all aglow and plumped up from increased circulation.) But remember your visor and sunscreen!

And, of course, walking regularly will help you to stay firmer and maintain a more youthful figure and posture—though many of us will be happier if we accept figures that are strong but no longer girlishly slim.

No, this program is about turning away from the mirror for a month and focusing on the world around you. In a fun, indirect way, you may gain renewed self-respect as you immerse yourself in things historic: statues, parks, or buildings that have stood the test of time and bring character and elegance to your neighborhood, town, or surrounding area. Granted, sometimes they need loving care and a face-lift, but historic buildings and homes have incomparable depth and intriguing stories to tell when you get to know them (just like you). Plus, you may feel more at home in your own community than ever before when you understand them better.

It's a good idea, too, to realize that focusing on negative images of aging can literally affect how you age. Negative stereotypes that we hold in our minds or keep on the tips of our tongues ("I'm getting old, wrinkly, senile; just call me a bag lady"—whatever you say to yourself on bad days, even jokingly) can even affect our walking speed and gait!

It pays to think of ourselves in more glowing terms, such as wise, strong, capable, and radiant. Pick the ones you like and substitute them when you find your mind wandering in the other direction.

## Aging, Memory, and Brainpower

Studies have shown that people who exercise regularly as they age perform significantly better on tests involving reason, memory, and reaction time. We know that by exercising regularly, even people in their seventies (and probably older) can improve their ability to do complex tasks and ignore distractions, which are the kind of mental abilities that allow us to drive a car, for instance. It all seems to have something to do with increased circulation, which probably cleanses and restores our central nervous system and floods the frontal lobes of the brain with increased oxygen. Exercise has also been shown to help alleviate depression and reduce the effects of stress, which can dim our "bulbs" significantly, too!

But another side to the equation is mental stimulation. I kept this quote from Gandhi tacked above my computer at work for several years: "Live as though you will die tomorrow, learn as though you will live forever." As we age, our brains do best if we stay actively engaged in learning. And as neurologist and neuropsychiatrist Jeff Victoroff, M.D., says in his book *Saving Your Brain* (Bantam, 2002), memory games and passive stimulation aren't enough. Active, energetic learning and teaching others what we've learned require the most from our brains and stimulate restorative growth. Exercise and active learning not only boost brainpower, they may protect us from Alzheimer's disease.

Learning about local history and architecture isn't just about learning dates and facts from another time. It challenges us to think about our present and our future as well. It makes us ask questions about what it was like to live during a certain era and how industry and technology have shaped our lives for better or for worse. With an active imagination, and with a personal history that now spans half a century, more or less, history comes alive for us in our fifties and beyond. We can suddenly make so much more sense out of it, relating to it in a way that was impossible when we were in junior high or high school—or even college. So if you slept through history classes when you were sixteen, don't let that deter you from exploring local history now. You may find a whole new world of meaning opening to you.

I've arbitrarily divided areas that might be of interest to you into three categories: historic landmarks and museums, neighborhood architecture, and historic cemeteries. That last category may shake you up a bit if you've recently been jolted awake at midlife like most of us are by the fact of your own mortality. But did you know that during Victorian times, cemeteries were considered serene places of beauty, full of flowers, sculpture, and poetry, and many townspeople found them perfect places for walking and Sunday picnics!

## Historic Landmarks

These can include statues, parks, ancient trees, buildings and houses, museums, churches, boats, commemorative plaques, living history villages—any place or thing that the culture has noted as remarkable by putting up a sign and telling you about it. Call the local library to find out if you have a local historical society. They most likely will be able to tell you what's available in your immediate area. You might also look up museums in your yellow pages. In my phone book, there are twenty-two listings. Of course, I live in a very historic area with many buildings dating back to the 1700s. Several of the historical societies are mentioned there. And I even discovered a museum I didn't know about at Mack Trucks, Inc. Now I'll have to go see it! Assemble pamphlets, check museum hours, and pinpoint the landmarks you'd like to visit on a map. It would be fun to post the map on a wall and share your destinations with friends and family.

If they happen to have ample ground around them, you may decide to drive to the sites, park your car, and walk the premises. If they're smaller landmarks, you can figure out a route that takes you on a pleasant walk around them or to and from a parking spot. I suggest wearing a pedometer and recording your step counts each day, rather than figuring out miles or tracking your time. You may be doing some pretty leisurely walking, but it's still a good idea to record your steps and give yourself credit for exercise.

If there are docents or tour guides of any kind, take advantage of their knowledge when you have the time and stroll around with them. They always have the most interesting stories, and you may even discover that you'd like to become involved with the organization and lead walks yourself. Sometimes that includes the fun of dressing up in costume. One of my future goals is to become a historic guide in downtown Bethlehem, Pennsylvania during the Christmas season, when visitors arrive by the thousands from all over the world. I can play dress up with a black cape and bonnet (and sneakers) and guide my group by lantern light while pointing out the historic buildings and giving a history of the Moravian settlers.

This is an opportunity to start a scrapbook, whether online or paper, with your comments, photos, and mementos. And be sure to keep track of the best walks that you might want to return to again and again.

## Architecture Appreciation Walks

Identifying varying styles of architecture in both new and old houses and other buildings is challenging and fun. It requires some study on your part. A beginner's guide called *What Style Is It?: A Guide to American Architecture,* by John C. Poppeliers, S. Allen Chambers, and Nancy B. Schwartz (John Wiley and Sons, 1995), is a pocket-sized guide that can help you decipher facades, windows, doors, arches, roofs, and other architectural details so that you can connect what you see to a style like Georgian, Federal, Colonial, or Craftsman. Even if you live in a community of mostly new homes, you'll be able to detect the influences of previous styles on modern-day designs.

I also recommend *Architecture for Beginners* by Louis Hellman (Writers and Readers Publishing, 1988) because it's funny and engaging, with its cartoon format and somewhat sarcastic style. Both these books are available used and new through www.Amazon.com and may be part of your local library collections. A more in-depth and detailed guide would be *A Field Guide to American Houses* by Virginia and Lee McAlester (Knopf, 1984).

Browsing through these books will make you more aware of things to look for: basic shapes, ornaments, windowpanes, roof lines, columns, materials (wood, brick, stucco, and so on). Trying to determine the style of house and the time in which it was built is like putting together a puzzle. For instance, if an old home has windows with many panes of glass, that could indicate that it was built before the 1800s, because until the nineteenth century, it wasn't possible to make the larger panes. If you see a regular, rectangular façade of brick with flat columns and marble trim, you might be looking at a house from the late eighteenth century of Georgian or Federal style.

You can learn interesting tidbits about the whys and wherefores of architectural details. For instance, the mansard roof (which you might see on a McDonald's as well as on a fancy or historic home) was invented in seventeenth-century France to disguise an additional story as a roof to avoid taxation, since property taxes were levied according to how many floors a building had.

Did you know that the little ornaments at the edge of slate roofs are sometimes called snowbirds? They do look a little like small wrens or house sparrows with wings spread. Their purpose is to keep the snow from sliding off the roof onto the sidewalk below as the roof begins to warm up under the winter sun.

### American Volksport Association Walks

The American Volksport Association (AVA) is the American branch of an international organization. There are clubs all over the United States whose main purpose is to create noncompetitive walking events for the public to enjoy. Many times, AVA walks, which are usually 6.2 miles long, center around an historic or culturally rich area. Some AVA walks are yearly or one-time events. Others are year-round events, called YREs. YREs can be done by anyone, anytime. You just go to the start point, pick up a map, and go. You can find out more about the AVA and all their walks and clubs by going to www.ava.org or by writing to them at AVA, 1001 Pat Booker Road, Suite 101, Universal City, Texas 78148. They also have an information hotline at (800) 830-WALK.

## Cemetery Walks

During the nineteenth century, cemeteries were not just isolated memorials to the dead, but gathering places for the living. Formal Victorian cemeteries were often well-designed landscapes full of monuments and sculptures, trees and flowers. Winding trails and picturesque views provided a perfect atmosphere for an afternoon stroll or a family picnic combined with a visit to honor departed family members.

Even more simple cemeteries provide solitude and interest for a walker. Gravestones tell their own stories with dates and quotes. Today it's uncommon to find many people in a cemetery unless they are there for a funeral. But in 1861, Laurel Hill Cemetery in Philadelphia had to give out tickets to control the flow of visitors. In one year they had more than 140,000! "The cemetery became a place of social gathering," says the Laurel Hill pamphlet, "a rural retreat for city dwellers, with an environment for meditation, inspiration, and cultivation of the arts."

Laurel Hill is now a National Historic Landmark and provides an excellent walking tour booklet for its arboretum, taking you past the graves of famous and wealthy Philadelphians. It's wonderful to see so many species of trees in their full glory, more than 150 years old. But even more modern cemeteries, like the one where my parents are buried in Basking Ridge, New Jersey, which doesn't allow any monuments, make for great walking in a parklike atmosphere, with winding trails, beautiful trees, few if any cars, and no dogs on the loose or bicycles whizzing by.

## The Stalking Historic Landmarks Walking Program

Use the chart on the next page to keep a list of the various places you have found that make good walking spots. Write the details down so that you have an index of various walks, the length of time (or number of steps) they take, and any special notes about them that may entice you there. Describe the starting point and route. Also note how much time it took to get to and from your destination, if you had to drive there.

At the same time, use the calendar provided to keep track of your daily walks, whether they're on your treadmill, around your neighborhood, or with friends at work. When you have the time and opportunity, schedule in a walk to an historic landmark, cemetery, or architecturally rich neighborhood. Your list will slowly grow to include dozens of interesting and rewarding walking spots that you can rely on to coax you off the couch and into another world of walking.

| | WEEK 1 | WEEK 2 | WEEK 3 |
|---|---|---|---|
| **Destination** | | | |
| | | | |
| **Route** | | | |
| | | | |
| **Steps** | | | |
| | | | |
| **Time** | | | |
| | | | |
| **Travel Time** | | | |
| | | | |

*Walk Your Way Through Menopause*

|            | WEEK 1 | WEEK 2 | WEEK 3 |
|------------|--------|--------|--------|
| **Destination** | | | |
| | | | |
| **Route** | | | |
| | | | |
| **Steps** | | | |
| | | | |
| **Time** | | | |
| | | | |
| **Travel Time** | | | |
| | | | |

# Hang with Your Grandchildren

**Consider this program if you**

- have established a regular walking program and understand from personal experience the benefits of consistent exercise;
- have grandchildren in elementary school;
- have an urge to put some energy into a good cause.

**What you'll need:** The energy and enthusiasm to effect change in your community. A personal computer (or access to one at your local library) and experience with using a step counter and counting your own steps would certainly be a plus, though not absolutely necessary.

## Grandmothers Can Step Up to the Plate

Before writing this chapter, I got out an old photograph of my first birthday. I'm sitting in the backyard with my mother, who is thirty, and my grandmother, who is about the age I am now, fifty-two. My grandmother has tightly curled, graying hair, wire-rimmed glasses, a matronly flowered dress that reaches to mid-ankle, thick stockings, and stocky, black orthopedic shoes. Though her face is not heavily lined, she has the appearance of being about seventy. Contrast that with how I look at her age, today. My hair is cut short, flecked with gold streaks, and spiked with gel. I'm wearing a pair of tight bicycle shorts for walking and a big Peter, Paul, and Mary T-shirt and sneakers. I have glasses, but they turn into sunglasses when I go outside, and I think they look pretty "cool" even though they are wire-rimmed. Of course, you can't *see* the bifocal lenses.

Grandmotherhood has changed quite a bit in the last fifty years. Many grandmothers today live to see their grandchildren graduate from college and begin to raise families. They are most likely working when their grandchildren are born, and they have active personal lives. They've experienced a revolution in women's rights, from simple things like being able to wear pants to school in the 1970s (I remember the day! Most male teachers remarked that they were relieved they no longer had to stand in front of a classroom of adolescent girls in miniskirts) to entering the job market in full force, breaking into many male-dominated occupations and assuming places of power in boardrooms, banks, and political arenas. The rocking chair image of grandmothers is quickly receding, or at least being pushed back about thirty years; now grandma is more likely to teach you how to water-ski than how to knit or crochet (though she may still help you bake cookies!). She may take you to the mall, play video games, buy you your first "kid's meal" with a toy, or fly with you to Disney World.

At first, I planned to write a program to help these women with grandchildren exercise in a meaningful way together. But the more I thought about it, the more I felt it would not have application for very many women. Unless you are in very close proximity to your grandchildren, and are not working full-time, you're probably not likely to have the time or energy to engage them in a regular walking program of any kind.

But I do believe that grandmothers can help their grandkids or someone else's children improve their chances for healthier, happier lives by helping to institute walking programs in the schools. You may have more time, confidence, or political clout than their mothers and fathers, who have so many responsibilities at this time in their lives that social activism resides very low on their "to do" list.

As I'm sure you know, physical activity has been doing a disappearing act in most school districts. When you and I were young, many of us walked to and from school—and even home for lunch! In addition, we had gym time for almost an hour every day. That was in addition to after-school activities like dance, baseball, football, softball, and scouts. We also played outside after school, after dinner, and most of the weekend.

Today's elementary school kids might have gym only once a week. They may be driven to and from school, even if it's only a short distance, because both parents are on their way to work. They spend more time watching TV, playing with computers, and competing with video games. Their most limber joint may be their thumbs!

Childhood obesity is rampant due to a lack of physical activity and the over-consumption of high-sugar, high-fat, highly processed foods. Most everyone is aware of this now. We learned on the nightly news that McDonald's hires child psychologists and uses child focus groups to determine how best to market their food to children and parents. Companies that promote questionable eating practices to children are being scrutinized and encouraged to improve their nutritional standards. The formaer Secretary of Health and Human Services of the United States, Tommy Thompson, has brought considerable attention to childhood obesity and the need for creative programs to improve the eating and exercise habits of both children and adults.

I am on the advisory board of The National Coalition for a Healthy America (www.forahealthyamerica.org). With the help of various partners, NCHA has developed two simple, turnkey programs for use in elementary schools. They are easy for teachers to implement and have been designed according to guidelines provided by the Centers for Disease Control. And they are the least expensive alternative out there that we know of, costing only about twenty-eight dollars per student, which includes a workbook, a pedometer, and access to online resources for tracking student results.

The program encourages both in-school activity and at-home activity so that parents can be encouraged by their children to be more active and eat more healthfully. (Kids can be very effective transmitters of this kind of information.) The program includes activities to increase awareness about the need for exercise as a lifelong activity and provides a way for teachers to get kids active during the school day. While many school gym activities tend to exclude or intimidate less athletically gifted kids, this is a program that includes everyone, regardless of size, speed, or coordination.

The program developers also give suggestions for fundraising in the local community so that costs to the school district can be minimized even further. In fact, there may be funding available to your community through one of their existing sponsors.

There are two basic programs: the I-Step Program and the Walk Across America Program. You can view them on the Web site. If you like what you see, you can contact NCHA for advice on the best way to approach your local school district or elementary school principal or PTA. (If you don't have access to a computer, call the group's toll-free number, (877) 843-2358.)

The program is very versatile and can be implemented for just one class, for a whole school, or for a walking club. As its popularity grows, there can be competitions between classes or grades or even between schools, with each child contributing to the total number of steps. To be good role models for the kids, teachers are encouraged to participate as well.

A few years ago, I helped three elementary schools implement a walking program sponsored by the local newspaper and local businesses. We kicked off the program by holding an assembly at each elementary school to introduce the program to the kids and generate enthusiasm. It was a simple program. The kids took some time every day to go for a walk around a measured course on the playground, lead by one of their teachers, and their mileage was recorded. There were a variety of incentives in place—stickers, little charms for a string bracelet, and pizza parties for the winning class-rooms and schools. The program was exceptionally well-received by students. Teachers were somewhat reluctant to add something new to their plates, but they found that the kids were better behaved, more relaxed, and even more attentive when they got their daily walks! So the teachers soon became avid participants. The kids were challenged to walk to a certain imaginary destination, but they far outpaced our expectations. And in the end, to our surprise, we found that the incentives were far less important to the kids than just getting outside and walking. Imagine that!

These programs do work; they can be effective in enhancing children's health and well-being and impacting an entire community. If you see a need where you live, be a mover and shaker in your area. It probably won't take a big investment of time or energy; it really depends on how involved you want to become. Your involvement may be as simple as introducing a teacher or an administrator to the program through a letter or an e-mail. If they like the program and want to implement it, but need more funds, you could get involved in creative ways to raise money. It's a little step that could have a major impact close to home. And you'll be a role model, too, because you've already established your walking program and others will see you walking every day in their neighborhood. You go, Grandma!

### Fun Walks with Grandkids or Kids of Any Age

There are two great walking-related activities that are engaging to all ages and are fun to do as a group. One is orienteering, which is a sport that involves following a terrain map to find a series of orange and white markers called controls. The controls have punches attached to them so that you can punch your card to show that you've found each one. It's sort of a well-orchestrated treasure hunt and requires stamina, map reading, and compass skills. You make your way to the finish line as fast as you can, if you're competing. But if you're just having a fun day in the woods, you can go at your leisure.

Orienteering is unique in that it has very competitive events where people run through the woods in a race to the finish while simultaneously holding events for beginner and intermediate participants. Rather than having to bush-whack through underbrush while reading a complex topography map, a begin-ner can follow a series of trails or pathways to find the controls. For more infor-

mation about orienteering events, go to www.orienteering.org. This is the international organization's Web site, and from here you can find your local organization's events and information.

Another fun activity that has become popular in recent years is called let-
terboxing. This involves following clues that lead you to a buried or hidden box
with a stamp, and it's another treasure hunt of sorts. It's a very informal game,
with clues posted on the Web site at www.letterboxing.org. Players are
encouraged to create their own personal stamps to imprint on the letterbox
notebook when they discover it. And everyone is encouraged to create his or
her own letterboxes and sets of clues to add to the growing number that are
buried throughout the country. I was surprised to find that there are several letterboxes hidden within a twenty-mile radius from my home.

# Nature and Gardens for Healing and Rejuvenation

**Try this program if you**
- are in need of any type of healing, whether it's physical, mental/emotional, or spiritual;
- have been feeling stressed, overworked, fatigued, or nervous;
- are looking for renewal in any area of your life;
- feel bored with your normal walking routine;
- are recovering from winter doldrums;
- are recovering from overuse of your treadmill.

**What you'll need:** A list of local parks and maps; books on historic gardens; a notebook to jot down the names of plants you might want to add to your home landscape (optional).

*"Nature doesn't bang any drums when she bursts forth into flower, nor play any dirges when the trees let go of their leaves in the fall. But when we approach her in the right spirit, she has many secrets to share. If you haven't heard nature whispering to you lately, now is a good time to give her the opportunity."*

*—from "Experiencing," Osho Zen Tarot: The Transcendental Game of Zen*

When I was a child, my parents often took my sisters and me to museums and estates where there were large and wonderful gardens. I remember being completely fascinated with them because of their winding paths and continual surprises. I loved walking in these gardens simply because they were *fun*. They seemed mysterious yet safe, beckoning you onward with every turn. What's around *that* bend in the path? I feel the same nearly half a century later.

Many of these gardens were done on a large scale, with dramatic plantings, sculpture, ponds, and private areas for conversation. They belonged to the nineteenth-century royalty of America, like the Vanderbilts and the DuPonts. I remember sitting alone on a cement bench by a small fountain, surrounded by fragrant roses, feeling as though I could hear the voices of people from another time whispering their confidences and laughing.

Modern scientific research has shown what ancient peoples, saints, poets, and philosophers have known for centuries: Natural areas and gardens are places where healing takes place. Horticultural therapists now bring the healing power of plants into hospitals and nursing homes where technological medicine had pushed nature to the wayside. Just the sight of trees through a hospital window is known to speed healing, reduce the need for pain medication, and reduce complications after surgery.

While it's wonderful to know that science can prove the beneficial effects being in nature has on our physiology, like lowered blood pressure and increased immunity, most of us don't need a scientific study to know that going for a walk in a natural area calms the mind, relieves tension, and restores our bodies to a more natural rhythm.

To take advantage of the restorative effects of nature, you only have to expose yourself to her beauty and bounty. Walking in parks, greenways, or botanical gardens will automatically help you to heal your body, mind, and spirit. You need only place yourself in nature's care by being present and paying attention.

I think you can experience a soul-soothing nature walk anywhere where your exposure to trees, grass, flowers and other plants, and water is greater than what you're generally exposed to, day to day. Any change in scenery perks up my mood and gets me to pay more attention to my surroundings. When I lived in downtown Allentown, Pennsylvania, in a neighborhood of townhouses devoid of trees, a walk in the suburbs felt like a wonderful garden walk. The lush lawns, landscaping, and garden plantings soothed my cement-weary eyes. Now that I live in an area that's somewhat rural, my "garden" walks are along the Delaware River and canal towpath. There, I feel completely enveloped in greenery, and the movement of the river and the glimmer of sunlight off the water add to my sense of peacefulness and of being a part of nature's flow.

Of course, nature doesn't have to be green to be healing—though my guess is that green trees have a more soothing effect than bare, gray ones when viewed from a hospital bed! I personally have a hard time with the world when November comes, the leaves are down, and no snow has fallen. Maybe it's a function of seasonal affective disorder (SAD) or just the sense of loss when the brilliant golden and red leaves have disappeared. But if I get out there and walk anyway, allowing the physical effects of exercise to boost my mood, I can usually find aspects of nature to revive myself too, whether it's squirrels scurrying up trees with acorns or more spectacular views of the river once the foliage lays the landscape bare. And I know that spring is hidden somewhere under those dry brown leaves, that the woods are not dead, but rather just resting and working on another level. It's a good analogy for when we feel dreary and "gray" in our own life cycles. Our creative energies may be percolating just below our conscious awareness.

## Going for the Green

Preparing for a four-week series of garden or greenway walks will take a little bit of research up front. I suggest the following:

- Contact your local recreation department and county parks department for a list of local parks and maps. Ask them specifically about walking trails or easy hiking paths.

- Check to see if there are any local hiking clubs. They are also a good resource for nature trails and may have scheduled walks you can join.

- Go to your local library and search for books on historic gardens. If you're not a good Web searcher, ask a librarian to help you search the Internet to locate possible botanical gardens or estate gardens in your area that are open to the public. (American Automobile Association Guides are also a great help in locating historic homes and botanical gardens.) Figure out how far you'd be willing to drive on a weekend or other free day to walk in a spectacular garden.

Here are a couple of my favorite books that have helped me locate wonderful garden walks near and far:

- *Gardenwalks: 101 of the Best Gardens from Maine to Virginia and Recommended Gardens throughout the Country* and *Walks in Welcoming Places* by Marina Harrison and Lucy D. Rosenfeld, two women who love to explore and have spent years searching out these wonderful places. Just be sure to call ahead to get updated information on hours and costs.

- *A Guide to the Sculpture Parks and Gardens of America* by Jane McCarthy and Laurily K. Epstein. Large-scale sculptures are all the more breathtaking in a natural environment. I find the combination of monumental sculpture, earth, sky, and a brisk walk far more thrilling than an indoor museum visit.

Use the calendar on the following pages to plan your healing walks. Find four wonderful greenways, gardens, or parks that can be your regular companions for the next four weeks. Return to the same location every day for as many days of the week that you feel able. If you can find something within walking distance of your home, all the better! There's a wonderful quote from essayist John Burroughs: "To learn something new, take the path you took yesterday." Getting to know a particular natural area is both enlivening and comforting. Each day that you go back to the same park or garden you are sure to see something new, something you missed the last time, or something that has changed, even if it's just the sky or the weather.

Save exceptional gardens, trails, or greenways that require a longer drive for your weekend walks. Take a Saturday or Sunday to yourself, or go on the walk with your spouse or a trusted friend. Make sure whomever you decide on for a companion is as interested in your destination and your walk as you are. You won't be doing much healing if you're worried about whether the other person is watching the clock or dragging their feet, literally or figuratively. Take a picnic in a backpack, along with some bottled water. And don't forget your digital camera; a computer slide show of your explorations is a nice way to relive your walk later in the week.

While there is much to see at some of these large gardens and estates, give yourself a chance to take a brisk walk around the property first, before you get tired from stopping and standing as you look at details of the garden or the landscaping more closely. Bring a notebook to jot down the names of plants you might like to add to your home landscape.

You may want to try a Breathwalk while walking, to clear your head from any negative thoughts or inner chatter. Or simply breathe deeply and focus on the beauty of nature around you.

If you have a partner, you might want to try an experiment I like to carry out with walking groups. I'll ask partners to hold hands and allow one of the pair to close their eyes and walk. People enjoy tuning into all the other sensations they've shunted to the background of consciousness—the smells, sounds, feelings on their skin, bodily perceptions of space around them, and so on. This can be a wonderful exercise for expanding awareness as well as feeling trust with your partner.

Another way to enjoy the day with a friend might be to agree ahead of time that your walk will be a kind of silent retreat. Sometimes when we walk with others, we just rerun problems and chatter endlessly in circles, making ourselves miserable or escalating our negative feelings, rather than releasing them. Or we feel we have to talk to be polite or entertain the other person. Agreeing up front on a few hours or even a day of silence can put both of you at ease with quiet and contemplation. And you may be surprised at the degree of communion you feel with each other and your surroundings.

Here are two more exercises that can help you reconnect with and feel a part of the natural world during a walk:

In *Reconnecting with Nature,* Michael Cohen, Ed.D., suggests focusing on your breathing, without changing it in any way. As you breathe out, imagine you can see the molecules of carbon dioxide flowing out of your nose and being absorbed by the leaves of the plants that you're walking by. At the same time, see molecules of oxygen flowing from the leaves of trees and other plants into your nose and mouth. There's no right or wrong way to experience the exercise. Just notice how you feel when you actively imagine this very natural process going on all around you. Another exercise you might want to try was suggested by Jack Borden, founder of For Spacious Skies, based in Lexington, Massachusetts. Jack, a former television broadcaster in Boston, had an "Aha" experience staring at the sky one day after a long hike near Thoreau's Walden Pond. He suddenly realized that most people don't pay any attention to the sky. He also noted that children often draw the sky at the top of a picture, as though the sky were above us; he realized that we don't think of ourselves as being "in" the sky. As you walk along a pathway, imagine yourself immersed in the sky, in the same way that a fish is immersed in the water. A fish breathes through its gills, taking in oxygen from the water that surrounds and supports it. You're taking in oxygen through your nose and mouth, surrounded by the air that supports your life. Notice how it makes you feel, as you walk along, to recognize that you are "in" the sky and supported by it.

If you are attracted to these kinds of exercises, you might like to take an online course called Reconnecting with Nature at www.ecopsych.com. It is a ten-week course that you take online with a small group of other people from around the globe. You experience a variety of exercises with nature, explore dreams, and share your experiences with the rest of the group via e-mails. The cost at the time of printing is $290. I took the course several years ago and enjoyed it very much. I hope to take it again and move further along in the degree program, using it to help people to connect with nature on my walking vacations and other classes.

And finally, another of my favorite nature teachers is Joseph Cornell, who became well-known through his first book, *Sharing Nature with Children,* which was published in 1979. I met Cornell at a private workshop and felt privileged to sit in the audience during two of his John Muir presentations in Pennsylvania, where he simply and elegantly portrayed the naturalist through first-person storytelling. His book *Listening to Nature* (Dawn Publications, 1987) is a series of photographs, inspirational quotes, and simple nature activities designed to take you into the heart of nature, rather than keep you on the outside simply naming and analyzing her many aspects. Cornell also wrote a pocket-sized book, *With Beauty Before Me,* which you can easily take with you on a walk. You can use it alone or share it with a friend or group.

After rereading several of Cornell's books, I decided to order a new one. I left the next day for a glorious hiking vacation in the mountains of southern Oregon and the redwood forests of northern California. When I returned, invigorated and refreshed by the experience, Cornell's book had arrived, and I opened it to this poignant quote from Muir:

> *"Climb the mountains and get their good tidings. Nature's peace will flow into you as sunshine flows into the trees. The winds will blow their own freshness into you, and the storms their energy, while cares will drop off like autumn leaves."*

I've created a four-week calendar with a special nature quote to reflect on each week. Approach this program with a gentle spirit. You are part of nature, and you should adapt the format to your needs and inclinations, your own natural rhythms. How long or how far you walk is up to you. As you immerse yourself in a natural area, you may find that your pace slows a bit, but that you walk farther than usual, drawn forward by the natural beauty around you and your own innate sense of adventure.

Choose a nearby walk for your busier days, and schedule a longer, more luxurious walk on weekends or whenever you have more free time. Record your thoughts, feelings, time spent, and the location of your walk. Use the exercises above or explore some of the tips found in the suggested books. You may even want to translate this program into a photo scrapbook, with your own additions of poetry and quotes.

# Week 1

*"Sometimes it seems to me I must just quit the city's din and dust, for fields of green and skies of blue."*

—Nixon Waterman, Far from the Madding Crowd

| | Thoughts |
|---|---|
| **Monday** | |
| | |
| **Tuesday** | |
| | |
| **Wednesday** | |
| | |
| **Thursday** | |
| | |
| **Friday** | |
| | |
| **Saturday** | |
| | |
| **Sunday** | |
| | |

# Week 2

*"I frequently tramped eight or ten miles through the deepest snow to keep an appointment with a beech-tree, or a yellow birch, or an old acquaintance among the pines."*

—Henry David Thoreau

| | Thoughts |
|---|---|
| **Monday** | |
| **Tuesday** | |
| **Wednesday** | |
| **Thursday** | |
| **Friday** | |
| **Saturday** | |
| **Sunday** | |

# Week 3

*"God is the experience of looking at a tree and saying, 'Ah!'"*

—*Joseph Campbell*

*"The wonder is that we can see these trees and not wonder more."*

—*Ralph Waldo Emerson*

| | Thoughts |
|---|---|
| **Monday** | |
| | |
| **Tuesday** | |
| | |
| **Wednesday** | |
| | |
| **Thursday** | |
| | |
| **Friday** | |
| | |
| **Saturday** | |
| | |
| **Sunday** | |
| | |

# Week 4

*"I only went out for a walk, and finally concluded to stay out until sundown: for going out, I found, was really going in."*

—John Muir

| | Thoughts |
|---|---|
| **Monday** | |
| | |
| **Tuesday** | |
| | |
| **Wednesday** | |
| | |
| **Thursday** | |
| | |
| **Friday** | |
| | |
| **Saturday** | |
| | |
| **Sunday** | |
| | |

# Birds! Birds! Birds!

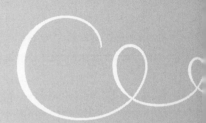

**Try birding if you**
- need more stimulation during your walks;
- feel the desire to appreciate nature and birds in new ways;
- love to collect or categorize;
- want to participate in environmental, conservation, or scientific initiatives;
- would like to have an outdoor activity to do with children;
- are looking for something to do with the binoculars someone gave you for Christmas a few years ago;
- enjoy meeting new people with a common interest.

**What you'll need:** A good bird guidebook, a decent (but not expensive) pair of binoculars, a notebook to record your sightings.

## Bird-Watching for Walkers

There are 51.3 million bird-watchers in the United States and more taking up the activity every year, according to surveys from the U.S. Fish and Wildlife Service. I consider myself a casual observer. I love watching birds at my birdbath and hummingbirds drinking nectar from my hanging fuchsia basket. And I enjoy carrying binoculars on walks and hikes and in my kayak, to get a better look at birds I might encounter along the way.

Many avid bird-watchers keep lists. They learn to identify birds by their physical features, markings, habitat, songs, and behaviors. Some people keep lists of the birds they see in their backyards. Some keep "life" lists, meaning they keep records of every bird species they have ever seen, and they'll travel to faraway places to expand their lists. Others may be less concerned with keeping lists and more interested in observing birds in the wild, enjoying a closer connection to nature that way. They may participate in annual bird counts, reporting to local conservationist groups.

Birding can be something you do alone, with friends and family, or with a special group or organization. Local Audubon societies or other birding groups (check with your recreation department or any bird-related stores in your area to find them) frequently plan group birding walks where you can learn a lot about identification from naturalists and ornithologists. The task can be somewhat frustrating at first, like any new sport or activity. Identification skills become stronger as you practice them. For me, just learning how to catch the bird with the lens of my binoculars can be a challenge!

Birding is associated with protection of birds, as well as appreciation. The Massachusetts Audubon Society, founded in 1896 by two prominent Boston women determined to stop the slaughter of birds for their plumage and feathers for fashion purposes, is one of the oldest and most influential conservation movements in America.

If you're contemplating becoming a birder, you might enjoy reading about the life of John James Audubon, the man whose colossal life work of searching out, painting, and publishing lithographs of birds resulted in the publication of *Birds of America* in the early 1800s. At the time, he sold his work by subscription, which cost $1,000. Today, an original copy sells for about $3,000,000. You can download a twenty-eight-page booklet about Audubon and his work from the Internet at www.haleysteele.com, for no charge.

Since I associated the name Audubon with the intellectual elite of Boston, I found it fascinating that John James Audubon was more eccentric, born in Haiti, the illegitimate child of a French captain and his chambermaid. His father took him to France, and he and his legal wife adopted Jean-Jacques at the age of four. At eighteen, Audubon was sent to take care of land his father owned in Pennsylvania in order to save him from the violence of the French Revolution. Free to roam the woods and countryside, Audubon became interested in hunting and sketching birds. Audubon eventually gained fame and fortune by painting birds in a lifelike, animated way. He did this by taking freshly killed birds and inserting wires in them so that he could position them for painting. Audubon's paintings were converted to lithographs that continue to be prized by American collectors, though initially his work was rejected in his own country; he had to gain success and notoriety in London before Americans began to appreciate his prodigious talent.

If you've never had more than a passing interest in birds, looking at Audubon's books or prints can help you to appreciate their awesome beauty and variety. Reading about the twists and turns of his life also reminded me how often our lives flutter between serendipity and tragedy before gaining a certain momentum later in life that can lead to new horizons. Audubon was in his forties before he started pursuing his painting and publishing efforts full-time. Reading about his life may give you inspiration to look over your own life from this "over the hill" vantage point, not with an eye to your successes or failures but to hunt for clues as to what interests, instincts, or passions you may have left behind that you can make time for now. Musing about these ideas on your daily walks can be highly creative!

For use on their birding walks and hikes, most people start with a Peterson Field Guide. Roger Tory Peterson was a modern-day naturalist who spent his life identifying, painting, and photographing birds. His guides help the birder by pointing out identifying marks and grouping similar birds together so that it's easier to make comparisons between birds that look alike. Most bookstores carry a variety of them, or they can be found at www.petersononline.com.

I happen to live in a prime area to observe hawks in migration. In my college days, we would drive out to the little-known Hawk Mountain Sanctuary in Kempton, Pennsylvania. We'd hike to various lookouts and rocky outcroppings in early September, hoping to catch sight of raptors passing through on their southern migration. Later, I learned that this is one of the premier places *in the world* to watch the migration of eagles, hawks, and falcons. Today, the Hawk Mountain Sanctuary is a world-renowned education and conservation center. About a year ago, I returned for a hike, the first in about eighteen years, and found several hundred people perched on the most accessible rocky ledge, armed with every size and shape of camera and telephoto lens. If you're willing to hike farther away from the main trails, though, you can escape the circus atmosphere and enjoy some solitude while observing the spectacle of the soaring hawks.

One nice place to observe birds with grandchildren is from a bird blind. You can sometimes find one at wildlife sanctuaries. It consists of a wall or enclosure that you stand or sit behind, looking out of slits or holes to observe birds eating at feeders. The birds can't see you, and you can often see a wide variety of species and behavior in a short amount of time. Combining your stationary bird-watching with a walk around the sanctuary makes for a very pleasant morning or afternoon. Of course, you can keep your eye out for the birds you've seen at the feeder, like a nature treasure hunt.

Binoculars are the one essential piece of equipment you'll need, in addition to a bird identification guide. When I was a kid, I used to lug out my father's World War II binoculars—big, heavy metal things—to follow the squirrels hopping from limb to limb on the oak trees that surrounded our house. Thank goodness we no longer have to hang something that heavy around our necks! I now have a lightweight pair that almost fits in the palm of my hand. I prefer to stuff them in a pocket, since any kind of weight seems to bother my neck, and besides, they clunk around on my chest when I'm hiking. There are some binoculars that are easier for people with eyeglasses to use; it has something to do with the distance your eyes can be from the lenses, and some magnifications make it easier than others for a beginner to bring a bird into view. More expensive varieties allow you to view greater detail from greater distances. Prices range from about $59 to hundreds of dollars. As you get more involved in the sport, the higher-grade binoculars become an added pleasure. There are videos to watch that explain birding basics, audio- and videotapes to help you learn birdsongs, and software for list management.

I caught Diane Porter on her cell phone, returning home from a morning bird walk. She and her husband own Birdwatching.com, a Web site that promotes birding and products for bird-watchers. They also write birding articles for publications like *Bird Watcher's Digest*, several of which are posted on their site. Diane was a bit breathless, hiking up a hill, as she shared her enthusiasm for this activity and cited her morning encounter with a bird she'd been looking for for months, perched on the berries of a sumac bush. "I didn't know they ate fruit," she said. "I'm going to go back tomorrow to see if they were really eating the fruit or picking the insects off."

"Birding can be enjoyable for innumerable reasons," notes Diane. "Some people just like the adventure of spotting birds; some like the competitive thrill of finding specific species and building lists. Others enjoy taking photographs or participating in conservation efforts or scientific investigations. Some people enjoy birding more in a group, while others prefer solitude in nature. And like me, many people interested in birding do some or all of these things!"

Diane noted that there are *some* bird expeditions that consist of driving from one location to another, the major exercise being getting in and out of the car. "I hate those kinds," she said. "Walking and hiking are definitely part of the pleasure and the spiritually restorative aspects of birding. Plus, it's a great sport for the mind. It's very mentally stimulating and requires learning and focus—a real mental workout!"

In the beginning, you can just start observing birds in your immediate environment—in your backyard or during walks around the neighborhood or through nearby parks. As you learn more about birds and their habitats, investigate birding books, or hook up with local birding groups, you may discover new places to walk, such as around lakes, through marshes or bogs, on nature trails, or in bird or wildlife sanctuaries. Natural areas that perhaps never seemed particularly inviting or interesting may suddenly seem like treasure troves as birding opportunities.

What follows is just a framework, a suggestion for kicking off a birding/walking program. Sometimes it helps to plan and schedule a new venture; immersing yourself in it will give you a better idea if it's something you'd enjoy pursuing.

## The 4-Week Beginning Birder Program

- Buy or borrow binoculars.

- Buy or borrow a bird guide for your area. Your local library should have plenty. Check to see if they have bird-watching videos you could review.

- Ask your local reference librarian for a list of local organizations that might have bird walks. Try to find at least one organized bird walk to join in on.

- Make a list of local natural areas that might have especially good bird-watching possibilities. Find a buddy to accompany you if you feel vulnerable in any location. Of course, birds can be found almost anywhere, but finding them in parks, pond areas, marshes, meadows, lakes, woods, and along rivers might be easier than spotting them in your neighborhood. (Plus, searching for them in these locations allows you some privacy. You might feel a bit awkward and look a bit suspicious using your binoculars near houses!)

### Week 1

Spend some time with your field guide. Make a mental note of the birds you know you've seen in your area. Get familiar with birds the book says might be in your area. Take the book and the binoculars out with you on your daily walk. Just get used to the idea of using them. Practice spotting birds with your binoculars. It's an art!

### Week 2

Make a point to attend a birding lecture, slide presentation, or birding walk in your area. Begin making a list of birds you've seen. Tack it on the refrigerator to remind you of your new hobby. If you don't have a birdbath, create one. It doesn't have to be fancy or expensive. Place it near a window so you can see it when you're having breakfast or dinner. Turn off the news, and commune with nature outside your window.

### Week 3

Plan a day hike with a friend or family member. Take your birding gear along with you. Stop every once in a while to listen to birdcalls, and try to spot birds in your surroundings with your binoculars. Buy a bird feeder and put it somewhere where you can see it; if you look out a kitchen window when you're standing at the sink, this could be a great spot for a feeder. I have a friend who has about ten feeders against a rocky backdrop and pine trees directly in front of her kitchen sink. It's awesome—like being at a bird blind.

### Week 4

Plan to walk at sunrise and sunset several times this week. That's when many birds tend to be more active and vocal. Use your ears as much as your eyes to take in their presence around you. Notice any changes in the way you feel about going out for a walk. Do you feel more anticipation, less reluctance? Do you spend more time walking, feeling more absorbed in observing nature than in wrestling with your thoughts? You may find this sport growing on you. As Diane Porter says, "Birding is a quest. You set out to see birds, but the prize you come back with can only be described as happiness. Learning to bird is like getting a lifetime ticket to the theater of nature."

Use the following month-long calendar to record your walking times, places, the types of birds seen, and your feelings during the walk.

| WALKING TIMES, PLACES, BIRDS, FEELINGS | | | |
|---|---|---|---|
| Week 1 | Week 2 | Week 3 | Week 4 |
| **Monday** | | | |
| | | | |
| **Tuesday** | | | |
| | | | |
| **Wednesday** | | | |
| | | | |
| **Thursday** | | | |
| | | | |
| **Friday** | | | |
| | | | |
| **Saturday** | | | |
| | | | |
| **Sunday** | | | |
| | | | |

# *Walking Vacation Preparation*

**Try this program if you**
- are ready for a wonderful travel adventure;
- need a reward or goal to work toward;
- enjoy vacationing in small groups with like-minded people;
- want to enjoy your active vacation without soreness or blisters;
- are not sure you're "fit" enough for daily walks or hikes of six to twelve miles.

**What you'll need:** A good pair of walking shoes and a good pair of off-road shoes or hiking boots (the type of shoe you should select depends on where you're going; ask your tour operator what she recommends for the terrain); a day pack that you feel comfortable wearing for hours.

On my very first walking and hiking vacation, I fell in love with this type of vacation. Never before had I felt so relaxed and at ease on a vacation. I loved meeting new people and sitting down to breakfast and dinner with an enthusiastic group that was eager to share themselves and their experiences.

Not having to plan, to make daily decisions, or to consult maps was another big plus. We got up in the morning and our guides would almost take us by the hand. All we had to do was enjoy the ride, the walk, the scenery, the food, and the company.

During my twenty-year stay at *Prevention*, I traveled this way almost exclusively as a single woman, and even after I remarried. My husband shared my enthusiasm for walking, hiking, and seeing new places. It was a relief not to have to negotiate what we'd do during a trip. Women recently widowed or who are unable to find travel partners find these kinds of vacations a great way to see new places, meet new people, and enjoy vacation time without feeling isolated or at risk.

I've walked and hiked in England, Wales, Switzerland, Austria, Puerto Rico, California, Vermont, New Mexico, North Carolina, Massachusetts, Virginia, Pennsylvania, and Oregon. And I have loved every single tour.

There are hundreds of companies that offer walking vacations today. In fact, after I left *Prevention*, I started my own travel company. You can view my trips on my Web site at www.walkforallseasons.com. I am slowly building a repertoire of destinations that focus on great walks without too much strenuous hiking, and that offer pleasing accommodations, cultural attractions, and excellent restaurants. In addition, I work with a long-established company, called Walking The World, which offers walking vacations for travelers "fifty or better."

This type of vacation seems to appeal mostly to the forty-plus market, with many energetic people in their sixties and seventies, even eighties. Many women are tentative about whether or not they have the stamina to accomplish a particular walking vacation. Don't be afraid to call and ask. A tour operator should be able to help you decide which, if any, of his or her trips would be suitable for your fitness level.

The better shape you're in, the more fun you'll have. It is important to prepare for these trips, as you will most likely be doing far more walking and hiking than you normally accomplish in a week. I've seen people suffer with blisters because their feet weren't sufficiently toughened, or because their boots were too new. I also had folks arrive for a trip crippled by heel pain, usually plantar fasciitis, because they tried to prepare but did too much, too soon.

So take some time and plan ahead for your trip. Set up a training program that will include getting used to any new gear, like walking shoes or hiking boots, carrying a day pack, and going up and down hills like those you will most probably encounter. Make sure you get a clear idea of the terrain you will encounter on your trip so you can adjust your preparation accordingly. Some trips consist of far more walking than hiking, and vice versa. Hiking is far more strenuous and will require some additional preparation, but the views you encounter are well worth the effort. On the other hand, I run a tour along the Delaware River and Canal that is entirely flat, easy walking, but also has wonderful views of the river and cliffs. It's a great trip for beginners at this type of touring.

Hiking or walking poles are invaluable on trips like these, and I highly recommend them. They can help you climb and descend hills, steady you when you're crossing water or rough terrain, and even just give you something to lean on for a good back or hip stretch. If you'll be scrambling over rocks or climbing rocky inclines, hiking poles with steel carbon tips will serve you much better than rubber-footed walking poles.

If you are going to be hiking, but you live in an area where the terrain is decidedly flat, I suggest any of the following: Work out on a stair-climber, if you have access to one; walk up and down the stairs in your house or workplace, to strengthen your legs; or find a stadium and walk up and down the stairs a few times, a couple of times a week. You'll also find the standing squats routine on page 178 very helpful in strengthening your legs for hiking.

When you walk to prepare for your vacation, wear the same shoes or boots you'll be wearing when you travel. Don't opt for a new pair of shoes or boots at the last minute. Even though they may feel heavenly in the store, it's too risky. On one trip in Switzerland, I had to use my pocketknife to cut away the tops of one woman's hiking boots that were rubbing her ankles raw.

You'll also want to make sure you have the perfect socks to wear with your shoes and boots, and buy extra pairs so you don't have to wear anything but what feels best. During your trip, it's a good idea to change your socks at lunchtime to avoid blisters. Powdering your feet to soak up moisture and cut down on friction can be nice, too. Also, pack your day pack with a few items to give it the approximate weight of what you expect to carry with you (poncho, camera, water, binoculars, and so on). Start wearing it on several of your preparatory walks and hikes every week.

Make sure you have rain gear that will both protect you and let the heat of your body escape. If it keeps you dry on the outside but makes you sweat on the inside, you're not going to feel very good in it. Most tour guides will take their groups walking in the rain, rather than sit back at the lodge. And on all-day hikes, you may simply get caught in a storm. Lots of people like big ponchos with hoods. I like ponchos but prefer a rain hat, so I can see and hear better. A breathable rain suit with pants is really great, but if you use it only once in a blue moon, it may seem like a big investment. I had a nice pink one once, made of Gortex, but I lost half of it in England!

What follows is a two-month calendar where you can chart your progress toward your walking/hiking vacation. If you're not already walking 30 minutes, most days of the week, then add a month to your preparation to get to that point. If you have any health concerns, particularly heart disease, diabetes, arthritis, or any musculoskeletal problems, *check with your doctor* before making your reservations.

One last tip: If you are flying to your hiking destination and will be changing flights, wear your hiking boots on the plane and have a change of clothes in your carry-on. I've had many occasions when people's luggage got lost and didn't arrive at their hotel for several days or more. While most people are happy to lend T-shirts and shorts, your hiking boots will be much more difficult to replace.

Your plan will vary depending on the duration and intensity of your particular vacation.

- Begin by increasing your daily walks by 15 minutes.

- At least two weeks before your trip, try to walk for an hour each day, five days a week.

- On the weekends (or whatever day is most convenient for you), plan some local hikes lasting from an hour to two hours or more, depending on your fitness level.

- If you live in a flat area, plan some 10- to 20-minute stair-climbing sessions, followed by a one-hour walk. Later progress to a two-hour walk.

- A week or two before your vacation, you might enjoy planning a whole day's walk—a mini walking vacation. Set out after a good breakfast, with a lunch and water in your pack, and wear your hiking boots. Walk for a couple of hours, break for a picnic, then set out for another couple of hours of walking or hiking. I've done this walking around local residential neighborhoods that have lots of hills. You don't have to go off to a faraway hiking spot. You'll feel very well prepared for your upcoming adventure, and you'll know whether your boots, backpack, or any other gear or clothing need adjustments.

|  | Sunday | Monday | Tuesday | Wednesday | Thursday | Friday | Saturday |
|---|---|---|---|---|---|---|---|
| TIME/ DISTANCE | | | | | | | |
| TIME/ DISTANCE | | | | | | | |
| TIME/ DISTANCE | | | | | | | |
| TIME/ DISTANCE | | | | | | | |
| TIME/ DISTANCE | | | | | | | |

|  | Sunday | Monday | Tuesday | Wednesday | Thursday | Friday | Saturday |
|---|---|---|---|---|---|---|---|
| TIME/ DISTANCE | | | | | | | |
| TIME/ DISTANCE | | | | | | | |
| TIME/ DISTANCE | | | | | | | |
| TIME/ DISTANCE | | | | | | | |
| TIME/ DISTANCE | | | | | | | |

# Chapter Three

# *Challenges of Midlife Weight Gain*

*I*'m not sure which is the greater challenge of thickening waists and flowering hips: reducing their size or learning to accept them. I know from experience that both are very difficult, and I don't pretend to have any perfect solutions.

Whether or not hormonal changes contribute to weight gain is not understood. Women complain of gaining weight *with* and *without* estrogen replacement. Though I considered myself pretty active most of my adult life, I gained *thirty pounds* in just one year during perimenopause. There are probably aging factors we don't fully understand yet that contribute to middle-aged weight gain. If I had to guess, I'd say a big factor for me has been becoming more sedentary overall, despite regular exercise periods. While I may walk for an hour a day now, more than ever before, and lift weights several times a week, teach yoga, ride bike occasionally on the weekends, and garden occasionally, I'm not as active, overall, as when I was taking care of two young children, running my household alone, walking kids to school and the dog around the block, running errands, and going to sports games after dinner.

So despite engaging in regular exercise of various types over the years, and a tendency to do active things with friends and family on weekends, like biking, skiing, playing tennis, kayaking, or hiking, I still gained weight at midlife. Having been thin most of my life (my nickname was Spider Legs Spilner in grammar school), I never imagined that weight would be an issue for me as I got older.

As the pounds added up, I began giving up things. I no longer ate bagels for a second breakfast when I came into work. I stopped eating doughnuts and baking brownies (except on very rare occasions). I switched to skim milk, whole wheat bread, and Egg Beaters. I rarely bought candy bars, and my husband and I agreed to keep peanut M&M's out of the house. I started cutting back on the Friday night pizza that had become a family ritual. I stopped eating cheese. We stopped having big pancake and eggs breakfasts on Sundays.

I probably tried every kind of diet suggestion, and then some. I ate low fat when that was the rage. I ate low carb. I tried the Peanut Butter Diet and the Ice Cream Diet. I joined Weight Watchers and then LA Weight Loss. I saw a nutritionist. After telling her about my eating habits and family history, she told me she wasn't sure if I'd ever be able to lose weight without taking an antidepressant. She felt my eating behaviors might be truly addictive—a way to boost serotonin levels in the brain. I didn't want to take antidepressants when I didn't feel depressed. I lost about eight pounds on her low-carb diet, but couldn't sustain it. I'm not saying I followed these programs perfectly and I still didn't lose weight. I'm saying I tried to follow them and *despite the best of intentions, I failed to stay with them.*

I even went to a hypnotist for several months after reading wonderful success stories in ads in the local newspaper. It seemed so simple. If I couldn't control my habits consciously, maybe I could control them *unconsciously.* According to the ads, once you underwent appropriate hypnotic training, you didn't even have to think about changing eating habits. They happened automatically. That sounded good to me, since calorie- or point-counting programs seemed to make me obsess about food. Apparently I wasn't a good subject. I got bored listening to the tapes day and night. And besides, the hypnotist was more overweight than I was, *despite* her good intentions. She ended up going on a European cruise where they did some kind of liver detoxification program that isn't legal in the United States. The last time I saw her, she did seem to be losing weight. But it didn't make me feel like continuing to invest hundreds of dollars in hypnosis sessions that didn't even work for her!

Various low-carb diets, like Atkins and South Beach, seemed effective initially, but after a certain amount of time, I'd crave the carbs, or a lack of time and planning would send me back to more familiar eating patterns.

As I was going through these programs over the years, and having to write articles with titles like "Walk Off the Pounds," I received many letters from women who were successful at losing weight. But I also received many letters from women around the country who said they walked and walked and could not drop a pound. They were frustrated voices I could identify with. But what alarmed me was that *because they saw exercise mainly as a way to lose weight, they seemed ready to throw in the towel when they didn't get the results they expected.* I found myself feeling the same way. An activity that I used to find extremely pleasurable was becoming a burden, a frustrating reminder that I was overweight, rather than a way to maintain my health and well-being. On some days, walking became more of a stressor than a stress releaser.

I realized I needed to change my attitude and help those frustrated readers change theirs. I corresponded with them by mail and e-mail and published their feelings in my newsletter. I encouraged them to keep walking, and to look to their eating habits, knowing just how difficult a chore that was! I asked them to see the major benefits of walking as better health, increased energy, stress reduction, and feelings of well-being, rather than mainly a way to burn calories. Eventually, reflecting on my own experience with controlling my diet, I encouraged them to accept and love their bodies as they were, and to focus on healthful eating and the benefits of daily exercise, rather than weight loss. Many wrote to me about their sense of relief, which seemed to stem from being given permission to accept their bodies.

I believe women who are moderately overweight are being made to feel far more at risk than they really are for future health problems. Not only do they feel frustrated because they can't return to their teenage figures or match the devastatingly slim images of beauty in magazines or on the big screen, but they feel guilty and scared because they believe their extra pounds are a *major health risk.*

Fortunately, research does not support that conclusion. The crucial factors that promote health are lifestyle factors, not readings on the scale. When people make efforts to eat healthfully and get active, they get real health benefits.

Edward Gregg, Ph.D., an epidemiologist for the Centers for Disease Control (CDC), analyzed data from 6,400 overweight and obese adults. He found that people who tried to lose weight, and did, live longer than people who don't try. But he also found that those who tried, but didn't lose weight, also lived longer. And while doctors know that losing just a little bit of weight can produce substantial health benefits, media and magazine images give the impression that if you're not skinny, you're a loser on all counts. Various weight indexes lump everyone together and give no credibility to differing body types. If you don't fit the numbers, you're considered fat.

Steven Blair, P.E.D., president and CEO of the Cooper Institute in Dallas, also feels we've put too much emphasis on the scale. He believes this diverts people's attention away from the more important goal—being active and eating healthful foods.

Today, I'm starting to let go of my "I'll be thin again someday" fantasy, and to accept the fact of my middle-aged body. I'm starting to give away clothes I've been saving for the future "Thin Me." And I'm shopping for clothes that flatter the figure I have *now*. I'm focusing on who I am now, appreciating my health and strength, and acknowledging my willingness to take responsibility for my health by my continued dedication to exercise, regardless of what the scale says. And I like to remember what Gurucharan Singh Khalsa said to me one day, when I revealed some of my frustration to him. "Now is the time to focus on radiance," he said, reminding me that as we age, we naturally lose certain aspects of youth and beauty, but our inner beauty continues to shine and grow. The rewards of my dedication to e xercise are not just a projected added year or two to my life span. I rarely get colds or the flu, even when my husband comes down with them. My blood pressure was 110 over 65 last week. My resting heart rate is about 55. Although my LDL cholesterol is somewhat high, my HDL levels are high, so my overall ratio is good. (And I've read enough about cholesterol readings to be skeptical of its value as a determining factor in heart disease.) I ask for the C-reactive protein tests to judge my vulnerability to heart disease, and they show positive results. And I seem to have overcome much of my vulnerability to back pain.

Am I saying that *you* should give up on weight loss? No, I am not. But I'd like both you and me to stop beating ourselves up over what the scale says or what magazines depict, or even what insurance tables say about our ideal weight. You need to know that as long as you stay active, your pre- or postmenopausal weight gain is not as much of a liability as you've been led to believe. Statistics and research tend to show that being active, eating well, and keeping a positive attitude go a long way toward protecting your health.

So what *should* you eat? A recent article in the *Washington Post* reviewed all the flip-flopping that has occurred in nutritional recommendations over the last ten years. You know the tune: "Don't eat eggs; it's okay to eat eggs.

Don't eat butter, use margarine. Oops! Margarine has bad stuff in it, go back to butter. Eat lots of low-fat pasta. No, don't eat pasta. Carbs make you fat." Need I go on? It's a wonder anyone listens anymore. But exercise advice has changed very little. It's good for you. Period. Whatever amount you can manage makes you better off than doing nothing at all.

Does that mean that I think we should all eat whatever we damn well please, whenever we want to eat it? I'm not saying that either. Eating conscientiously is important to your health, and the health of the environment. The quantity and quality of the foods you eat can help you stay healthy and feel energized. When I cut back on carbohydrates like bread, sweets, potatoes, and pastas, I feel much more energetic and can maintain concentration and focus for longer periods of time. When I eat more fruits and vegetables, I feel lighter and my digestive system works more effectively. When I buy organic produce, I know I'm voting with my dollar for a cleaner, safer environment. When I buy milk and beef from pasture-fed cows, I know I'm supporting the small farmer and helping to preserve that way of life and open space in my community. When I buy eggs from free-range chickens, I know I'm voting for healthful, humane animal husbandry.

Here's what I strive for when it comes to food practices:

**Eat whole, natural foods as much as possible.** That means fruits, vegetables, fish, poultry, beans, nuts, meat, eggs, and milk. As one nutritionist said to me, "If you can pick it from a tree or a bush, dig it out of the ground or shoot it, you can eat it." I would add dairy products to that list. I favor them. If you want to learn more about the importance of wholesome, whole-fat dairy products and traditional food practices, I highly recommend Sally Fallon's book, *Nourishing Traditions* (New Trends Publishing, 1999, 2001). A cookbook that explains the nutritional value inherent in traditional food preparation methods, *Nourishing Traditions* is also an exposé of modern farming and processing methods. There is scorching testimonial against the manipulation of food and nutrition research by powerful interest groups in the past fifty years that has led to the mass marketing of prepared foods that no one should be eating. I buy raw milk from pasture-fed cows from my local health food store, who gets it from a local farmer. I don't want the small farms in my area to disappear. I also make an effort to buy from farmer's markets, roadside stands, or grocery stores that buy from local farmers.

*Avoid processed foods, white sugar, white flour, hydrogenated oils, and products with high fructose corn syrup.* They either have no nutrient value or they are actually harmful to your health. Check labels. High fructose corn syrup is in just about every fruit drink and sweet processed food item. Some experts believe it contributes to the fattening of Americans because it is so prevalent and because it bypasses our sensory equipment for satiety. This means that we don't feel signals for fullness, so we just want, and eat, more.

Recently, a major health study involving more than 50,000 nurses was released that showed that women who drank one regular (not diet) soda or sweetened fruit juice a day gained much more weight than those who drank just one a month. In addition, their risk of developing adult onset diabetes was increased by 80 percent.

*Buy whole grain foods such as brown rice, 100 percent whole grain breads, and whole grain pastas.* Sprouted grains have even more nutritional value. The fiber of whole grains helps to make you feel full and helps regulate blood glucose levels, so you don't feel hungry again as quickly as you do after eating processed grains and flours. And fiber will actually help move some of the calories out of your system before they have a chance to be added to your fat stores.

*Watch your portions.* If you get the chance, rent the film *SuperSizeMe*. Americans are offered unbelievably large portions when they go out to eat. Often I can divide a plate I get in a restaurant into two or *three* meals. At home, use a smaller plate. Savor your food. Get more variety on your plate. Add more veggies and fruit, which will give you extra nutrients and fill you up with their fiber. If you're about to help yourself to seconds, see if you can wait twenty minutes, so you get a chance to feel satiated. Finally, pack up extra food and store it in the fridge before you sit down to a meal, so you won't pick at it.

*Drink water in preference to any other beverage.* Liquid calories really mount up fast, and most processed beverages are essentially junk food anyway. Experts recommend getting six to eight cups of water a day, which can include teas and coffee.

*Get enough calcium.* The recommended daily intake for postmenopausal women is 1,500 milligrams a day. The best way to get it is from natural sources, because the mix of calcium and phosphorous in dairy products is easily absorbed and perfect for your bones, but few of us get enough that way. So figure out how much you normally get from food and supplement the rest. One serving of dairy, like milk or yogurt, usually has about 300 milligrams of calcium.

**Take a good daily multivitamin as an insurance policy.** According to Fallon and many others, even our produce does not contain the nutritional punch it once did, due to modern farming practices, storage, and so on. A good multi should have 100 percent of the Daily Value of most nutrients. Once you stop menstruating, you no longer need additional iron supplementation.

**Buy fresh, local produce whenever possible.** Buy organic if you can afford it. If you can't, wash your produce carefully with a natural cleanser like Veggie Wash. Frozen produce is better nutritionally than canned, and it often has less added salt or sugar. I buy tree-ripened fruit whenever I can. What's the use of buying a peach if it never ripens and it tastes like sawdust? I grow my own tomatoes in my flower garden every year because it is just so easy. I put in two plants and always have some tomatoes to give away. If I see a local corn stand, I buy some and have it that evening. It's easy to fall out of love with fresh foods if they're tasteless due to too early picking or sitting around too long. One of the reasons I think we like Twinkies and other junk foods is that we know exactly how they will taste, every time.

**Stick to healthy oils like olive oil, flax oil, avocado oil, and coconut oil.** These oils cut down on inflammation, pain, and swelling and may also protect against cancer. Butter is acceptable. In fact, according to Fallon, raw butter from pasture-fed cows is high in CLA (conjugated linoleic acid). CLA encourages muscle buildup and helps prevent weight gain. You can find out more about this from Fallon's book and from the Weston A. Price Foundation. Visit www.westonaprice.org, or write to Weston A. Price Foundation, 4200 Wisconsin Avenue NW, Washington, DC 20016.

**When the urge strikes you, eat the highest-quality, least-sweetened, darkest chocolate you can find.** I find that a few squares of this type of chocolate will do what a whole bag of M&M's cannot. Chocolate is high in antioxidants that fight aging, and the carbohydrates found in chocolate boost serotonin, which elevates mood. Recently it was discovered that chocolate makes your arteries more flexible, though that's not an excuse to eat so much that you gain weight.

*Instead of focusing on foods you can't have, try to find foods you love that are healthful.* Try to be organized enough in your shopping habits that you have a continuous supply of healthful foods on hand. When we're really hungry, it's easy to eat anything in sight. Have fruits and vegetables washed, cut up, and ready to grab from the fridge. Make fruit and vegetable smoothies in your blender. (A recent concoction I made up on a hot summer day consisted of cantaloupe and pineapple, with a little crushed ice, whizzed in my blender. It was really refreshing! I used canned pineapple, packed in water.)

*Be gentle with yourself.* Enjoy your food. You don't have to be perfect. Your body doesn't have to be perfect. Your food doesn't have to be perfect.

# Special Bonus Yoga Section

The power of aerobic exercise to improve your health and your sense of well-being is well-documented. But there is another kind of exercise that is recommended by health experts, including the surgeon general of the United States, and that's what is known as "resistance" training. I laugh whenever I read that term. Most American women don't need training in *resistance*. We resist exercise just fine without any help or training. Of course, resistance training refers to building muscle mass and strength, and it's important because as we age, our muscles get weaker and smaller, both from natural aging processes and from lack of activity. Loss of muscle leads to a lower metabolic rate (we burn fewer calories every day, so we gain weight), weakness, lack of balance, poor joint support, falls, and eventually, an inability to take care of ourselves as we age.

Walking will of course lead to increases in strength and endurance, and since it is weight-bearing, it helps prevent osteoporosis. If you walk with poles or upper-body strength-training devices, like the Powerbelt, you'll get upper-body conditioning and some increased muscle mass, too. Strength training with hand weights, bands, or exercise machines is another option, and one that I revert to from time to time because of my need for variety and stimulation. But for all-around conditioning, strength building, and flexibility, and the added benefits of deep breathing and a sense of peace and inner calm and integration, I prefer yoga.

I experienced my first yoga class thirty years ago, when I was twenty-three. At the time, I can't say I got much out of it. I was strong, thin, and naturally flexible. Lifting my legs up and touching them behind my head in Plow Pose was a cinch. At the time, I was more curious about yoga philosophy. It would be another fifteen years before a back injury and increasing stiffness brought me to the yoga mat with a real appreciation for its power to soothe, center, and heal the body and mind.

I began taking yoga more seriously as a physical practice after spending a week in the hospital with a herniated disk. Pain and suffering are potent motivators! Studying with videotapes and books, I learned a variety of poses to help strengthen and stretch my back and hips. Often, I'd roll out of bed with a back spasm that zapped me when I stretched and yawned first thing in the morning, slither to the floor, and practice Cat and Dog Pose and Child Pose to stretch and soothe the spasm away. I found Downward Facing Dog to be a great way to fully stretch my calves and hamstrings when battling the heel pain of plantar fasciitis (the inflammation of tissue running along the bottom of the foot, causing sharp pain in your heel when your feet hit the floor first thing in the morning). If you have a dog or a cat, you'll see them do this natural stretch several times a day, after they've spent a long time lying still or sleeping.

In my midforties, I took a class for women who were going through perimenopause. It focused on restorative poses for deep relaxation and for opening the hips and relieving congestion in the pelvic area. We learned some inverted poses, where your head is lower than your heart; these moves are known as "cooling" poses, and when practiced regularly, they may help relieve the intensity and frequency of hot flashes and night sweats.

In my late forties, after going through menopause, I decided to enroll in a yearlong teacher training course that would give me a better understanding of yoga from the inside out. I figured the course would be beneficial for a book idea I was developing with famed yoga teacher Lilias Folan.

The book deal fell apart, but I continued with the training. I learned many different breath control techniques (called pranayama) and spent hours learning about yoga philosophy. I studied the yoga sutras of Pantanjali, which explain the ethical concepts that were originally part of all yoga training: nonviolence, action instead of reaction, gentle self-discipline, focusing on the present moment, attaining a peaceful state of mind, replacing unhappiness with joy, etc. Gradually, all the pieces of the puzzle came together, and time spent practicing the asanas (poses) made much more sense. As I observed myself and my reactions during my practice and in class, I learned so much about the way I approached my life—my tendency to push too hard, too soon; my lack of patience with myself; and the ways I constantly compared myself with others. I noticed a myriad of details about my personality that were really helpful, and I began to understand that practicing postures entails far more than simply stretching and strengthening the body.

We also explored and practiced a variety of meditation techniques that helped to calm and focus the mind and induce a deep sense of relaxation and peace. I believe this plunge into yoga training was pivotal in helping me get through one of the toughest years of my adult life. My mother, suffering from a rapidly progressing dementia, needed much care and attention. Another close family member suffered a serious depression. I was working full-time, running to another state sometimes twice a week, trying to find better than adequate care to keep my mother in her home, and at the same time deeply concerned while I watched another family member struggle with unrelenting sadness. I felt like I had leapt from "empty nest syndrome," when my two sons left home for college, headfirst into "the sandwich generation," where I found myself feeling squashed like wilting lettuce. My yoga training and practice helped me take care of myself while I helped take care of others. I'm not sure what I would have been like or felt like without it. Four months after my teacher training ended, my mother passed away while I calmly held her hand. I was calm and accepting in a way I never expected to be in such a situation.

Other benefits included increased flexibility, better range of motion, and a greater feeling of agility and suppleness. I gained greater strength in my legs and found that after a winter of doing just yoga, I could walk up the steep hills in my neighborhood that spring without stopping to gasp for breath as I normally do after being holed up for several months. Another surprising benefit was stretching away adhesions that had formed after some surgery on my neck. For several years, I had the annoying feeling of having a tight bandage wrapped under my chin. My surgeon had emphasized massaging the area vigorously after the surgery, but it was really painful and maybe I didn't do it enough. I'd given up on expecting the sensation to go away, but after about six months of daily yoga practice, where I was often stretching the neck area while lifting my head in easy back bends, like Cobra Pose, I noticed that the tight feeling was greatly relieved!

Compared to weight training, yoga leaves me feeling strong and supple rather than strong and constricted. Recently, I ran into a personal trainer with whom I had worked for several months a few years ago. She's my age and an accomplished bodybuilder. She told me she had recently started taking yoga and wished that she'd done so years ago because it made her feel so much more comfortable in her body!

## Not a Religion

Yoga is not a religion, as some people suspect, but an extremely practical ethical system that includes meditation, breathing techniques, spiritual ideals, and the practice of physical postures to help unite body, mind, and spirit. While the postures alone can certainly help you to enjoy better health, greater flexibility and strength, reduced tension, and a host of other health benefits, I do encourage you to read books, take classes, and watch videos that will broaden your perspective on this ancient tradition. (See the appendix on page 190 for some recommendations.) As our bodies change and age, and our lives go through seismic shifts in work and family life, not only the postures, but the whole attitude of yoga can help us to reorient our lives to what's important to us and to where we want to direct our energies, our love, and our passion in the future.

In the following pages, I will be approaching yoga primarily from the physical aspects. Presented here are postures that I found particularly helpful as a walker. When I was younger, I seemed to get along just fine without really stretching much. And I rarely entertained the idea of lifting weights. But at fifty-two, the more I stretch, the better I feel. And strength training, through yoga or other means, is a gift I give myself for an active, adventurous future.

### Finding a Yoga Teacher

Until the last few years, anybody could teach yoga, and plenty of people did it without any real training. Today there is a national certifying body, The Yoga Alliance, that can help you find a teacher who has at least a minimum of 200 hours of formal training or the equivalent. You will see the designation RYT after an instructor's name, which stands for Registered Yoga Teacher. I belong to The Yoga Alliance, and the group requires that I continue to learn, teach, and train in order to continue to receive my RYT membership card. To locate a registered teacher or studio in your area, go to www.yogaalliance.com or call (610) 777-7793. You can also e-mail info@yogaalliance.com or send them a self-addressed, stamped envelope at 122 West Lancaster Avenue, Suite 204, Reading, PA 19607. Or check with teachers in your area to see if they are registered.

## Ocean-Sounding Breath

Proper, deep breathing is a great physical and emotional cleanser. The reason aerobic exercise is so enlivening is that it forces you to breathe more fully and deeply than you normally breathe when you aren't active. Simply getting more oxygen into your brain cells helps you to think more clearly. As you do yoga, or meditate, you can learn to deepen your breath naturally while you are at rest. Many people have restricted breathing patterns due to tension, fears, anxiety, or, simply, bad habits.

Until someone taught me proper breathing techniques, yoga seemed like just another "gym" class to me. When I finally learned how to breathe properly, I found a whole new dimension of ease, integration, and opening. I remember, for instance, going to an early evening yoga class after spending the day battling the effects of a decongestant I'd taken early in the morning. I had been feeling very "spaced out," unable to concentrate, and *fuzzy* headed—and had pretty much tried to find things to do at work that didn't require too much of me. I came to the class hoping to relax and prepare for a good night's sleep. I was amazed to find that after forty minutes of focused breathing and poses, my mind seemed to reconnect with my body and I felt perfectly focused and alert. I remember feeling so surprised by it, because I had suspected that the class would merely put me to sleep.

While there are many different forms of pranayama that have particular effects on the mind and nervous system, *Ujjai* Breathing, also known as Ocean Breath, is one of the forms that is used concurrently with your yoga postures, and it's my favorite, all-around soothing breath. I teach it first thing in all of my classes. Below are the benefits associated with Ocean Breath; the list shows clearly why you may feel more focused and alert when you combine Ocean Breath with your yoga postures, or just practice it while seated.

- Relaxes the body and calms the mind

- Increases concentration by using the sound of the breath as the main focal point

- Induces a meditative state as you focus on the sound of the breath

- Stimulates circulation, metabolism, and blood flow, and increases energy

- Opens the alveoli in the lungs, allowing better oxygen absorption

Unlike other, more vigorous forms of yogic breathing, there are no contraindications with Ocean Breath, except that it should not be done after recent abdominal surgery.

The technique is pretty simple, though it may take some practice to get comfortable with it. When you are doing Ocean Breath correctly, your breathing sounds like the rise and fall of ocean waves, as if you were listening to a conch shell. When you use Ocean Breath during your poses, you can make it a bit more active and vigorous to help open your body and relax places where you are holding more tension or muscular tightness.

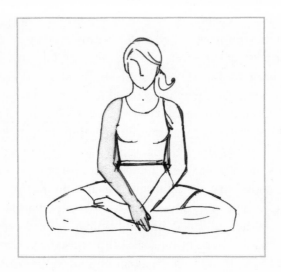

## Try It Now

1. Sit in a straight-back chair or on the floor with your legs crossed. Or you can practice Ocean Breath while lying down. Keep your spine comfortably erect.

2. Begin taking long, slow, deep breaths with your mouth closed.

3. Keeping the breath relaxed and gentle, contract the back of your throat slightly, creating a slight but steady hissing sound as you breathe both in and out. It is as if you are drawing your breath like a bow across the back of your upper palate, creating a soft but audible whisper of breath. Some compare it to the breath you make when fogging a mirror with an open mouth. (To experiment, hold an actual pocket mirror in

your hand and fog it with your breath. Then close your mouth and try to create the same feeling.)

4. Lengthen the inhalation and exhalation as much as possible without straining or creating tension anywhere in your body. Keep your breathing smooth and continuous; don't hold the inhale or the exhale.

Beginning your yoga sessions with a few moments of Ocean Breath can help you to calm your mind and let go of the anxiety, worries, or excitement of the day. This allows you to focus on your body and become more aware of how it works. Focus and concentration are important for many reasons, but especially so that you can stay attuned to your body's needs and avoid injury.

## My Favorite Yoga Poses for Midlife Walkers

When starting out, you may find that there are just a couple of yoga poses you want to practice regularly because they help you with some particular area of discomfort. You may not have a "practice" where you go to the mat every day; instead, you may simply stretch wherever you find yourself. If you become more involved, you will want to round out your program so that you have poses that balance your entire body. In any given session you will want to include poses that move your body into flexion or extension (forward bends and back bends); those that move your body into a lateral stretch, from side to side; and those that stretch your body by twisting to the left and to the right. Standing poses focus on lower-body strength and balance, while certain floor poses increase abdominal strength or strengthen the back.

The following are poses that I've found particularly helpful and are a perfect complement to daily walks. Walking tightens the hamstrings, hips, and calves, which can lead to various types of discomforts and injury; yoga can stretch out these areas and ease any discomfort. Many yoga poses may seem familiar because they have been incorporated into stretching routines for runners, walkers, and other athletes. If you are in the midst of perimenopause and suffering from hot flashes and night sweats, you should know that many yoga poses have a relaxing, tranquilizing effect. Those poses where your body is inverted may be particularly helpful.

Never force or strain at yoga. Be gentle with yourself. Move slowly in and out of poses with attention, so that you have the opportunity to make adjustments or changes before you injure yourself. Don't force. Remember to breathe continuously, and consciously relax into poses. You will find it an interesting challenge to maintain the strength required to hold certain poses, while simultaneously learning to relax any muscles not directly involved. This can be very helpful in everyday life because we tend to progressively tighten muscles inadvertently as we go about our daily tasks, such as driving, typing, and cleaning .

Yoga may open up a whole new world to you. I encourage you to attend some classes and get some hands-on instruction with a registered teacher. Videotapes and books are also very helpful. I've included some recommendations in the appendix on page 190

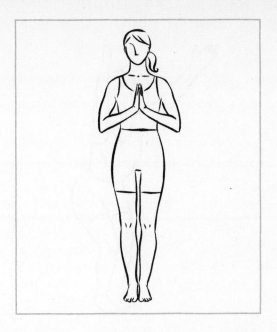

## Mountain Pose

Mountain Pose helps you focus intimately on all aspects of good, strong posture. As you learn to know your body in Mountain Pose, you can return to better posture in any situation in life or simply throughout your day and walk taller and more at ease. You will feel grounded, secure, and balanced.

Stand with your feet slightly apart. Feel the bottoms of your feet and shift your weight toward your toes and then back toward your heels, noticing the difference in your balance and posture. Then find the most comfortable spot, centered over your arches. Keep your knees soft, not locked. Locking your knees pushes your pelvis out of alignment.

Drop your pelvis into place by pressing your navel toward your backbone as you press your tailbone toward the ground. Notice the subtle shift. If you tend to be swaybacked like me, stand in front of the mirror as you do this, and notice how your protruding belly disappears! Lift your sternum slightly, being careful not to arch your back. Let your shoulders drop down, hands quietly at your sides. Bring your head into alignment with your shoulders as you press the top of your head toward the sky, lengthening your spine. Soften your gaze and breathe Ocean Breath for several breaths. To reorient your posture, practice Mountain Pose any time you find yourself standing in line. It's great to spend a moment in Mountain Pose before you walk, reminding yourself to stay tall and balanced.

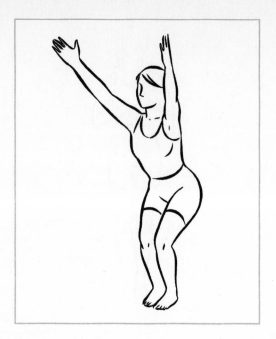

### Standing Squat Series

This series really strengthens your quadriceps muscles (thighs) and helps with climbing hills. If you have knee problems, be very careful with form; you may want to practice just the first or first and second positions and hold them longer, rather than squatting all the way down in the third position. If you're not strong enough to keep your balance, position a chair to one side or use a wall. Even a light touch on a stable object can make a big difference.

Stand with your feet about hip-distance apart. Find a place to focus on in front of you, to help with your balance. Raise your arms in front of you, straight out, parallel to the ground.

Sit back, as though you were going to sit down in a chair, and hold for several breaths.

Return to standing, then come up on your toes and sit again, this time keeping your back straighter. Go only as deep as feels comfortable. Hold for a few breaths and return to standing. Now bring your thighs and knees together for support and come up on the balls of your feet, then squat as far down as you can, keeping your back straight. Take a few steady breaths and return to standing. Release your arms.

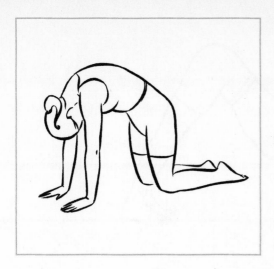 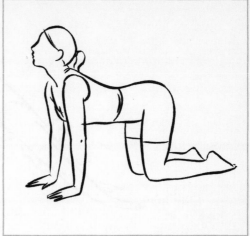

**Cat/Cow**

This was a primary yoga posture for me during the years that I suffered from almost chronic back pain. It eases early morning back stiffness and helps to relieve nagging sciatic pain. My chiropractor loves to tell the story of how his back went into a painful spasm at Home Depot while he was reaching for some plywood boards. When that happens, as I well know, you can feel as though someone has shot you in the back and you need to fall to the floor to take any weight off your back. He immediately went down, then rolled onto his hands and knees and began practicing cat/cow, much to the dismay of store employees, who wanted to help him up. "Just leave me alone for a minute," he said. The spasm released and he was able to walk out of the store.

Go down on your knees and place your hands on the floor, fingers spread. Try to make your back flat, with one unbroken line from tailbone to tip of head. Exhale and arch your back like an angry cat, bringing your belly button toward your backbone as your tighten your abdomen. Your head drops toward the ground and your tailbone curves down and forward. As you inhale, drop your belly down toward the floor, lift your head, and lift your tailbone. Inhaling and exhaling at your own steady pace, move back and forth between these two positions. You may wish to release by pushing your buttocks back to your heels, arms outstretched in front, to stretch and release your back. You may also want to roll onto your back and bring your knees to your chest, rocking side to side for a soothing lower-back massage.

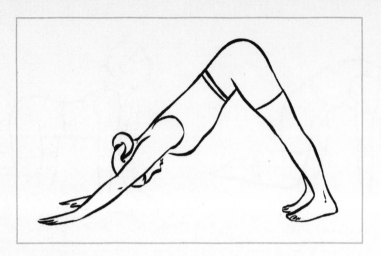

## Downward Facing Dog

Several years ago, when I asked Suza Francina, author of *The New Yoga for People over Fifty*, to name some of the best poses for walkers, this was her most recommended pose. It stretches the entire body from fingers to toes and helps open the chest and reverse rounded shoulders. It increases blood circulation to your brain and may stimulate the bones in your upper body to retain calcium, which may help prevent osteoporosis in those areas. Walkers will appreciate the stretch to the calves, which helps prevent heel pain and plantar fasciitis.

You should have a nonslip surface, like a yoga mat, to practice this pose. Begin on all fours, as in cat/cow pose, but place your knees slightly behind your hips. Place your hands slightly in front of your shoulders and spread your fingers, placing your weight on the fleshy part of your hand rather than the wrist. Curl your toes under on an exhale and straighten your knees, pushing your bottom toward the ceiling. Raise your heels high off the floor to try to get your buttocks even higher. Push yourself away from your hands, like you're pushing the floor away. Begin lowering your heels to the floor. If they feel very tight, alternate pushing one heel, then the other, toward the floor.

Breathe smoothly and naturally. Relax your neck and let your head hang down toward the floor. Spread your shoulder blades apart. Take several deep, even breaths. Release by returning to all fours. You may wish to push back, placing your buttocks on your heels and bringing your head to the floor in a puppy stretch.

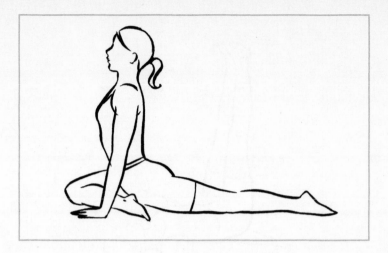

## Pigeon

Lilias Folan taught me this pose in my living room, when I asked her for a pose to help stretch out my tight hips for walking. Not only does it stretch the hips beautifully, but you'll feel the psoas muscle stretch on the opposite side as you press upward from your fingertips. You may want to place a pillow under your hip for support.

Start from a kneeling position. As you inhale, slide your left leg back behind you, toes and heel in alignment, knee to the floor. Shift your weight to the right and bring your right buttock to the floor, or place a cushion under it—many people, including me, will be too tight to get the buttock to the floor! Bring your right foot in front of your left hip.

Exhaling, lower your torso toward or over your thigh. Take several Ocean Breaths as you rock side to side, gently opening your hip.

Placing your palms or fingertips to the floor on either side of your forward knee, press into the ground and lift your torso to a vertical position, pressing down into your hips, arching your back slightly, opening your chest, and pressing up through the crown of your head. If you can't reach the floor with your hands, try placing them on top of your thigh.

Release your torso, bring your left leg forward, and return to a kneeling position. Then practice the pose on the opposite side.

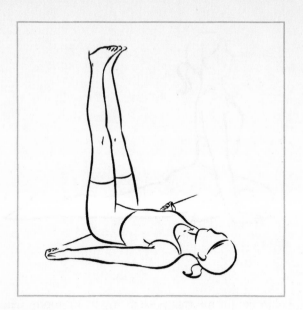

### Legs-up-the-Wall Pose

This is another pose Suza Francina recommended for me when we met at one of *Prevention*'s Walker's Rallies years ago. My only regret is that I don't do it enough.

My legs tend to swell during the day, and after a long walk my right foot is very swollen, due to an ancient injury. I also have varicose veins, which started appearing in my late teens or early twenties when I was waitressing. This pose helps reverse the flow of blood and reduces swelling. It's also very calming and restorative.

This pose is also a very safe way of doing an inversion. Since I am not comfortable practicing headstands (I am simply too concerned about hurting my neck), this is my way to get that gravity-reversing benefit. If you have heart, neck, eye, or hernia problems, you should check with your doctor before doing any kind of inversions, but according to Francina, people with mild hypertension can actually benefit from Legs-up-the-Wall as it tends to normalize blood pressure.

Begin by positioning your bottom sideways, to the wall. Then, as you roll back onto your elbows, swivel your body so that your feet come to the wall. Lay back flat on the ground and extend your legs up the wall. Wriggle around until your back and legs are comfortable. If your hamstrings are really tight, you may have to push your bottom several inches from the wall before you feel relaxed. Stretch your neck out along the ground, and position your head so that it is not tilted up, chin to ceiling, but aligned with your forehead. Allow at least five minutes to relax. You may enjoy covering your eyes with an eyebag or a soft, rolled-up towel.

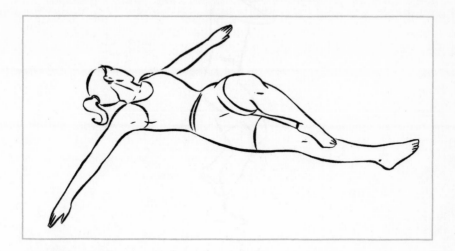

## Knee Down Twist

As I've aged, I've lost flexibility in my lower back and neck. This affects my ability to twist and turn and is surprisingly handicapping for me in several ways. Before I started taking yoga, it was getting more and more difficult for me to back up my car. I didn't even think about playing golf, and playing tennis would often set off a back spasm. Just plain reaching for things, as well as working in the garden, became more difficult. There are many forms of spinal twists, but this is one of my favorites because it is easy to relax into. If you practice racewalking form, this twist is a great way to stretch out your torso after all those hip rotations.

Lie on your back, with your knees bent. Focus on your back as you slide your right leg out straight, being careful not to allow your back to overarch. Place your arms straight out to your sides, palms down. Place your left foot above your right knee. Keeping your shoulders on the ground, allow your left knee to roll toward the right, toward the floor. Allow your left hip to come up off the floor as your torso moves into a gentle twist. Keep breathing deeply into the stretch. When you're ready, bring your back flat to the floor, release your left leg, and straighten it. Bring your right leg up and twist to the opposite side. Finish by rolling onto your flat back again and bringing your knees to your chest to release any tension in your back.

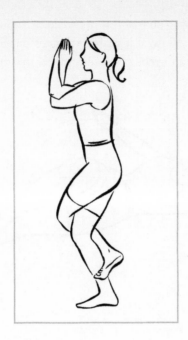

## Eagle Pose

Stretching out the upper back can be difficult to do. Long hours of typing, driving, or any activity we do out in front of our bodies, plus tension or anxiety, make us vulnerable to upper-back stiffness and pain. Then when we go for a walk and we finally get some circulation into the upper back, we can feel achy and uncomfortable. Eagle Pose is a great way to stretch that area.

Stand with your feet together or slightly apart. Raise your arms out sideways, palms down, like an eagle about to take flight. Let your arms swing toward each other, passing the left under the right. Then curl the left hand back in an effort to place your palms together. Probably the most you'll be able to do is catch the bottom of your palm with your fingers. That's a start. As you press your palms together, or fingers and palm, you'll feel your back open up. Play with this pose, moving from side to side, up and down, stretching out little corners here and there.

In the more complete pose, you go from here into a balance pose by standing on one foot and wrapping one leg around the other, keeping the knee of the standing leg bent.

Then stand up and release the leg and arms and approach the pose with the opposite arm and leg on top.

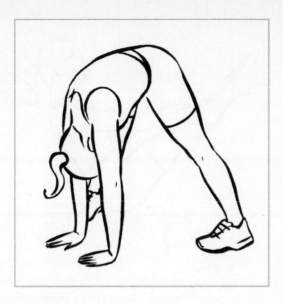

**Wide Angle Forward Bend**

All walkers need to stretch their hamstrings, and there are many ways to do that. But this is one of my favorite ways, because it feels so good and it's so relaxing. The lengthening of the hamstrings is gentler in this pose than in seated forward bends or forward bends with the legs together. I almost feel like I could fall asleep in this pose, it's so relaxing.

Stand on a nonslip surface and step or jump your feet apart; they should be parallel but turned inward slightly. You want a fairly wide stance, so you can reach the ground at least with your hands, if not your head. Place your hands on your hips and press down, lengthening your spine as you press up into the crown of your head. Hinge forward from your hips, keeping your back long and straight, and your knees soft, not locked, until your back is parallel with the ground, then fold all the way forward, releasing your hands toward the ground. You may want to place a block or firm pillow or folded blankets on the ground so that you can rest your head on them. You can simply rest your hands lightly on the ground. Or, for more stretch in your back, fold your arms and let the weight of your folded arms gently stretch you. Stay here for several breaths as you feel your back lengthen and your hamstrings release. When you're ready, I suggest bending your knees slightly to protect your lower back and then placing your hands on your hips and either sweeping your upper body back to standing or rolling up slowly. Bring your feet back together.

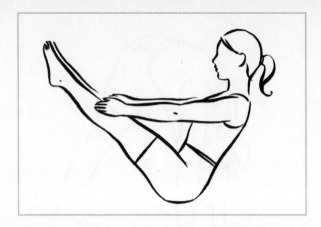

## Upward Boat

There are some poses I enjoy doing less than others. Often those are the ones I need to do the most! Upward Boat is one of those, because it requires strong abdominal muscles. Strong abs help you to maintain a taller, more aligned posture when you walk. When I practice this pose regularly, it's easy to see the difference in my ab strength. When I let it go, it's easy to see how fast I can lose ground in this area!

Sit on the floor, arms hugging your bent knees. Focus on keeping your back straight, pushing up through the crown of your head as you press your sitting bones into the ground. Rock back until you find yourself balanced comfortably on your sitting bones, back straight, not rounded, and release your knees, feet above the ground. Keep your knees bent as you reach your arms straight out in front, parallel to the ground. Steady yourself by keeping your abdominal muscles contracted, while remaining as relaxed as possible through your neck, shoulders, and legs.

If this position is easy, you can extend your legs from your bent knees. A more advanced position is to extend your legs upward, unbending your knees completely. Hold for several breaths, and release.

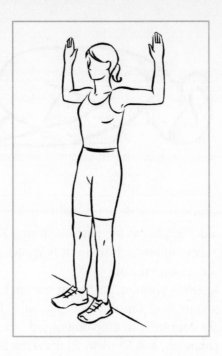

### Arms up the Wall

This isn't an official yoga pose, but an exercise I learned from the wonderful book *Back Care Basics: A Doctor's Gentle Yoga Program for Back and Neck Pain* by Mary Pullig Shatz, M.D. It helps to counteract a rounded upper back and shoulders, opens the chest and shoulders, and helps make it possible to bring your neck back into alignment. So many women have forward heads from doing desk or computer work. Just trying to bring your head into alignment isn't easy when all your muscles have become accustomed to holding it out in front. Walking with a forward head puts strain on your neck, shoulders, and upper back and can tire you more quickly. Good posture makes for a youthful-looking walk.

Stand with your back and buttocks and shoulders against a wall, heels a few inches away from the wall. Bring your arms up against the wall, elbows bent at right angles, the back of your hands touching the wall. (If you can't reach the wall with your hands, get as close as you can without straining.) While trying to keep your hands and elbows on the wall, slowly and gently raise your arms upward, straightening your elbows, then slide them back to their original position. To avoid arching your back, press your belly button toward the wall.

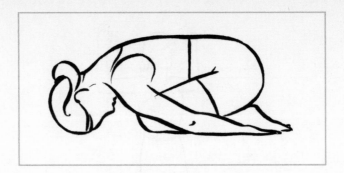

### Child's Pose

This is a wonderful pose to use anytime during a yoga session to relax and revive or to relieve lower-back strain. It is known as an anxiety reducer and may help lower blood pressure.

From a kneeling position, push your bottom back to rest over your heels as you bring your head forward to the ground. Push your thighs apart to allow room for your belly to drop downward, if needed. Bring your arms to your sides, palms up, and let them relax on the floor. Spend a few minutes breathing quietly. You can also use some folded blankets positioned in front of you, to support your upper body and head, and turn your head to the side, in Supported Child's Pose.

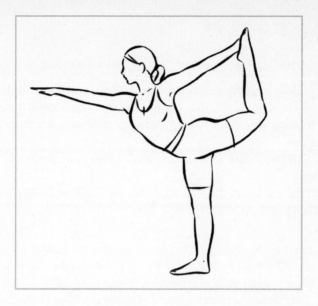

**Dancer**

Anyone who walks or hikes a lot knows that the quadriceps muscle (front of thigh) can become very tight. The traditional quadriceps stretch consists of bending the knee and grabbing the foot behind. Dancer is a variation of that kind of stretch, but it requires even more balance, which strengthens the little muscles in the lower legs and ankles. It's more difficult, but the added concentration and grace it requires make it both fun to do and more physically rewarding. If you're too tight to reach your foot with your hand, try using a strap so you don't strain your back or your leg muscles. Feel free to use a chair or table in front of you for support, as you gain strength and balance.

Stand in Mountain Pose. Bring your left arm straight up, palm facing forward, fingers together. Find a place to focus your gaze on the floor, out in front of you. Shift your weight onto your left leg. Lift your right foot behind you and grasp it on the side with your right hand. (Or loop a strap around it) Press your right foot back into your hand (or the strap). Bend forward at your hip, keeping your back arched, pressing up through the crown of your head as you look straight out at your extended arm. (You may wish to place your hand on a chair or table in front of you.) Breathe deeply as you press your right hip down, bringing it into alignment with the other hip.

When you're ready, release the leg as you bring your torso back to a standing position. Repeat on the other side.

# Resources

The market is flooded with books and videos on yoga. I suggest you go to a local bookstore (your library may not have a very current collection) and browse. There are so many approaches to yoga that you'll need to look and see what appeals to you right now.

Some books are very picture-based, others contain lots of explanation and philosophy.

Here are some of my favorites that are excellent for beginners as well as more seasoned yoga practitioners:

## Books

*The New Yoga for People over Fifty: A Comprehensive Guide for Midlife and Older Beginners* by Suza Francina, Health Communications Inc., 1997.

Contains detailed descriptions of poses as well as the use of props to make difficult poses accessible to beginners. Lots of great stories from women who came to yoga late in life.

*Yoga and the Wisdom of Menopause: A Guide to Physical, Emotional, and Spiritual Health at Midlife and Beyond* by Suza Francina, Health Communications, 2003.

Detailed information on poses that support the transition through perimenopause and menopause. More great stories from real people. Lots of helpful prop suggestions.

*Yoga: The Spirit and Practice of Moving Into Stillness* by Erich Schiffmann, Pocket Books, 1996.

Schiffmann gives the most sensitive, accessible, sensual descriptions of what yoga practice means and how to accomplish poses. For example, in his introduction, he writes, "The purpose of yoga is to facilitate the profound inner relaxation that accompanies fearlessness. The release from fear is what finally precipitates the full flowering of love."

*Practicing Yoga Postures: An Easy to Use Workbook* by Connie Weiss, Lurie Lane Publishing, 1991.

This is a great book for beginners who are trying to grasp how to put together a workout after attending various classes and never being able to remember what to do at home. Contains line drawings of postures in a workbook format that allows you to cut the pages and create a balanced workout page you can use at a glance.

# Videos

Yoga videos are great, and you really can come back to them again and again without getting bored. I have several easy ones for days when I feel stiff, injured, or out of shape. I also have more challenging ones for when I'm feeling supple and energized. Here are some of my favorites:

*Gentle Kripalu* with Carolyn Lundeen.

Two complete sessions. Great instruction. Gentle on the body. Slow moving, easy to follow.

*Back Care Yoga* with Rodney Yee.

This workout uses a chair as a prop. On days when I am stiff from airline travel, golf, or lifting something too heavy, or whenever my back and legs feel stiff, I love this workout. It gently eases me into stretches from the chair, then goes on to supported standing poses and floor work. He does go a little fast, though. Feel free to keep the remote handy and stop the program so you can breathe your way into a stretch at your own timing.

*Yoga for Weight Loss* with Suzanne Deason.

I can't vouch for the weight-loss part, but it is a great workout. Plus, it's very wonderful to see several sizes of women doing this yoga routine, with modifications in the postures to help you adapt.

*Lilias! Target Toning for Beginners* with Lilias Folan.

Now well into her sixties, the woman who brought yoga to television in the 1970s is still very active teaching and creating videos. This is one of many that I have tried. In this great video for beginners, Lilias walks you carefully through each move without making the explanations esoteric or complicated. Comfortably paced.

# Mats, Straps, Props, and Clothing

These are resources I have used. But there's been an explosion of yoga commerce online, and any Internet search will yield many discount houses and a wide variety of yoga equipment and clothing suppliers.

www.huggermugger.com

www.gaiam.com

www.thewalkerswarehouse.com

# Acknowledgments

I would like to thank Sara Donovan, walker extraordinaire, who directed the publisher to my door, Holly Schmidt at Fair Winds Press for following that lead and Donna Raskin for her editorial support and upbeat review of my work, and to my copy editor Amy Kovalski who remembers all the things I never can about grammar and punctuation and catches and slips of the keyboard (or my brain!)

In addition, I would like to acknowledge the continuing support of my friend and walking teacher, Elaine Ward, whose dedication to the sport of walking and racewalking is truly inspiring. Thanks to Jane Serues for including me in First Strides for Women in 2004. Thanks to my sister, Paula Spilner, PhD for helping me flesh out my ideas on architectural walks and for spending a blisteringly hot afternoon exploring Victorian cemetery pathways, and to Tom Rutlin, who continually inspires me to remember my walking poles! I'd also like to thank my long time friend, Gale Maleskey, R.D. who reviewed my chapter on weight-loss and nutrition and is always ready to hear what project I'm on to next. Thanks to my two Williams Township walking buddies, Dot Hagenbuch and Anne Beidler, who met me on the track or the road all summer long, making sure I was walking my talk while meeting my deadlines. And to my sons, Eric Spilner Schmitt and Robin Spilner, for still finding time in their busy lives to walk and hike with me.

And finally, thank you Dave, for being steadfast in believing in me and what I can accomplish and patient with my moods and frustrations. And finally, a pat on the head to Puppy, who never tires of being my walking pal and assures me I never have to walk alone.

# About the Author

*Maggie Spilner* began writing about walking for health and fitness as an editor for *Prevention* Magazine. She wrote booklets, newsletters and a monthly column for 17 years. While at *Prevention*, Spilner directed the Prevention Magazine Walking Club and ran their walking tour program, where she had the opportunity to spend time walking ancient pathways in England, Switzerland and Wales, as well as hiking trails around the United States.

Spilner received training in Dynamic Walking from Suki Munsell, PhD, founder of the Dynamic Walking Institute in Corte Madera California, where she became a certified trainer. She is also a certified Breathwalk Instructor, a registered yoga teacher, and studied massage therapy at Health Options Institute in Northampton, PA. In 2003 she won a National Journalism Award from the American Podiatric Medical Association.